Praise for

RESTART YOUR HEART

"This wonderful book explains for patients what physicians know about the important public health problem of atrial fibrillation. Dr. Desai is a cardiologist with special expertise in this area, and he presents clearly to patients what they should know about this problem in order to better guide and understand their many options available for therapy. Dr. Desai clarifies complex concepts with easy-to-understand language and provides an important perspective for patients. This book is a must-read for anyone who has atrial fibrillation."

–Kenneth A. Ellenbogen, MD, Martha M. and
Harold W. Kimmerling Professor of Cardiology,
Chair of Cardiology, VCU School of Medicine

"In *Restart Your Heart: The Playbook for Thriving with AFib*, my former colleague at the University of Chicago, Dr. Aseem Desai, a veteran specialist in the treatment of patients with heart rhythm disorders, tackles the epidemic of atrial fibrillation by going straight to the patient. He provides expert advice beyond what patients will find in brochures and other patient-education materials, and beyond what most time-limited encounters with physicians and other health care providers can offer. This book empowers patients who often have a lifelong condition that can put them at risk of stroke, heart failure, and disabling symptoms."

–Bradley P. Knight, MD, FHRS, Chester and Deborah Cooley
Distinguished Professor of Cardiology, Northwestern University,
Director of Cardiac Electrophysiology, Northwestern Medicine

"Dr. Aseem Desai is not only one of the most caring people I know, but he is unrelentingly dedicated to his life path by taking the time to write this groundbreaking book that is the defining word in overcoming AFib. In *Restart Your Heart*, Dr. Desai skillfully becomes a master teacher and guide who lets you know with uplifting simplicity how anyone can reclaim their life. This book is a gem."

–Cathy Lee Crosby, actress, producer, star of film, television, and stage, author of *Let the Magic Begin*

"Dr. Desai has written an excellent and comprehensive book on AFib focused on the patient. The book is accurate, well written, and well illustrated. It distills complex information in a way that patients can understand. I am especially impressed with the many patient stories, which increase the impact of the book and make it easier to read."

–Hugh Calkins, MD, FHRS, FACC, FAHA, FESC, Professor of Medicine, Johns Hopkins School of Medicine, Director, Johns Hopkins Cardiac Arrhythmia Services and Electrophysiology Laboratory

"This is a lucidly written book by an experienced expert and succeeds in empowering the patient. It has meaningful content and nice illustrations that will be very useful for any patient with this arrhythmia. The information is also highly relevant for the loved ones who support the patient."

–Kalyanam Shivkumar, MD, PhD, FHRS, Professor and Director, UCLA Cardiac Arrhythmia Center and EP Programs, David Geffen School of Medicine at UCLA

"The premise of *Restart Your Heart* is to help you overcome AFib on your own terms. It includes explanations of the condition and treatments, resources for dealing with the emotional impact of AFib, and touching stories. This very practical guide is full of great charts and compelling explanations for anyone living with AFib."

–Mellanie True Hills, CEO and Founder, StopAfib.org, author of *A Woman's Guide to Saving Her Own Life*

"In this age of information, books such as *Restart Your Heart: The Playbook for Thriving with AFib* are vital in order to get reliable information and recommendations. In this book, Dr. Desai gives us up-to-date knowledge from an experienced physician, as well as wisdom from his own personal experiences. He speaks to our heads as well as our hearts and skillfully brings in the connection between mind, heart, and body. He discusses beneficial tools that may not be presented in the typical medical visit, such as mindfulness, nature, and music. Anyone who has been given a diagnosis of atrial fibrillation, their family members, and practitioners alike will benefit from reading this book. It empowers patients living with atrial fibrillation to thrive and gives practitioners a valuable tool to educate their patients."

–Sheila Patel, MD, Chief Medical Officer, Chopra Global

THE PLAYBOOK FOR **THRIVING WITH AFIB**

RESTART YOUR HEART

ASEEM DESAI, MD, FHRS

Foreword by David Baker,
President and CEO of the Pro Football Hall of Fame

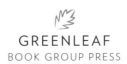

GREENLEAF
BOOK GROUP PRESS

This book is intended as a reference volume only, not as a medical manual. The information given here is designed to help you make informed decisions about your health. It is not intended as a substitute for any treatment that may have been prescribed by your doctor. If you suspect that you have a medical problem, you should seek competent medical help. You should not begin a new health regimen without first consulting a medical professional.

Published by Greenleaf Book Group Press
Austin, Texas
www.gbgpress.com

www.draseemdesai.com

Distributed by Greenleaf Book Group

For ordering information or special discounts for bulk purchases, please contact Greenleaf Book Group at PO Box 91869, Austin, TX 78709, 512.891.6100.

Design and composition by Greenleaf Book Group
Cover design by Greenleaf Book Group
Illustrations by Samantha Stutzman

Publisher's Cataloging-in-Publication data is available.

Print ISBN: 978-1-62634-708-3

eBook ISBN: 978-1-62634-709-0

Part of the Tree Neutral® program, which offsets the number of trees consumed in the production and printing of this book by taking proactive steps, such as planting trees in direct proportion to the number of trees used: www.treeneutral.com

Printed in China on acid-free paper

20 21 22 23 24 25 26   10 9 8 7 6 5 4 3 2 1

First Edition

For Lindsay, Oliver, and Chasey-Bear

CONTENTS

List of Illustrations xi

Foreword. xiii

Preface xvii

Acknowledgments xxiii

Introduction 1

STEP 1: BE INFORMED

Chapter 1: Cause. 15

Chapter 2: Confirmation 59

Chapter 3: Control 83

STEP 2: BE PREPARED

Chapter 4: Breathe 137

Chapter 5: Build a Toolbox 143

Chapter 6: Build a Team 157

STEP 3: BE IN CONTROL

Chapter 7: Be Watchful 163

Chapter 8: Be Updated 169

Chapter 9: Be the Master. 175

Conclusion. 179

Case Studies 183

Glossary 193

Bibliography 197

Index. 201

Notes 213

About the Author 215

List of Illustrations

Figure 1:
Blood Flow in the Heart   17

Figure 2:
Cardiac Conduction System   19

Figure 3: Individual Heartbeat   20

Figures 4 and 5: Heartbeat's Effect on the Ion Channel Receptors and Ion Channel Receptors Analogy   22

Figure 6a:
Arrhythmia Mechanisms   25

Figure 6b: Atrial Flutter Circuit—Ablation—Atrial Flutter Analogies   28

Figure 7a:
Types of Atrial Fibrillation   31

Figure 7b: Prevalence of Atrial Fibrillation and Projected Number of Patients   33

Figure 8:
Risk Factors of Atrial Fibrillation   43

Figure 9:
Triggers of Atrial Fibrillation   52

Self-Assessment:
AFib Risk Factors   53–55

Self-Assessment:
AFib Triggers, Figure 1   56

Self-Assessment:
AFib Triggers, Figure 2   57

Self-Assessment:
AFib Triggers, Figure 3   58

Figure 10: Holter Monitor   67

Figure 11: Event Recorder   70

Figure 12: Telemetry Monitor   71

Figure 13: Patch Monitor   74

Figure 14: Subcutaneous Implantable Monitor and Wireless Base Station   76

Figure 15: Smartphone-enabled Monitor and Apple Watch EKG   78

Figure 16:
Summary of Rhythm Monitors   80

Questions to Ask Your AFib Specialist, Part 1   81

Questions to Ask Your AFib Specialist, Part 2   82

Table 17:
AFib Antiarrhythmic Drugs   89

Figure 18: Cardioversion   92

Figure 19: Single-Chamber Pacemaker/ Dual-Chamber Pacemaker   95

Figure 20: Leadless Pacemaker/ Biventricular Pacemaker   96

Figure 21: AV Node Ablation   99

Figure 22a:
Types of 3-D Mapping Catheters   102

Figure 22b: 3-D Mapping during AFib Ablation   103

Figure 23: Cryoballoon Ablation and Radiofrequency Ablation   105

Figure 24:
Robotic Catheter Ablation   107

Figure 25:
Convergent AFib Ablation   108

Table 26: Rate Control Drugs   111

Figure 27:
Stroke Prevention: Screening   114

Figure 28:
Stroke Prevention: Treatments   116

Foreword

At the Pro Football Hall of Fame—the most inspiring place on earth—in Canton, Ohio, we assess greatness and calibrate excellence every day. After all, it's not the "Hall of Very, Very Good." It's the Hall of Fame, and it stands for *excellence.*

In the history of this great game, we estimate that there have been well over 300 million young men—and now women—who have played the game of football. There are only 5 million who have played it in college. There are only 29,000 who have played, coached, or officiated it in the National Football League. And as of this writing, there are only 326 people—181 of them living—who have bronzed busts in Canton and Hall of Fame "Gold Jackets," signifying those who represent a gold standard in their sport. That is *elite.* That is *excellence.*

Every year during "Selection Saturday," on the eve of the Super Bowl, I have the enormous privilege to knock on the doors of four to eight of the greatest ever to play the game and welcome them to Canton as enshrinees to the Pro Football Hall of Fame. It's easy to assume they fell out of bed "great" each morning and were simply born stronger, faster, and tougher than anyone else, but in reality, they each fought to be great. They persevered and overcame countless adversities. In the business of football, excellence is a battle that is fought over a long period of time. It is snot coming out of your nose, blood flowing from your lip, and a filthy uniform. It is having coaches with a game plan to follow over a sustained period of time, carrying an athlete and a lot of other people to a place of excellence and greatness. Most of all, each of these great competitors had *heart*—a heart for their city, their teammates, their coaches, their fans, and the game.

But if your heart is not healthy, it can change everything. I know from personal experience. I have faced atrial fibrillation. I've been short of breath, out of energy, weak, and sometimes dizzy. It has affected how I've felt, my relationships with others, and the work I do. When I first encountered this adversity, I attacked it the way we always do in football: I sought out the best "coaches" possible. I was fortunate to have in California an intelligent, compassionate, and competent cardiologist who recommended an incredible cardiac electrophysiologist. Together with my personal physician and cardiologist in Ohio, my team of coaches tailored a care plan that not only helped me return to good health, but also helped me perform at my best at all times. They not only restored my quality of life and all the loves of my life, but also my life's work.

In his groundbreaking book, *Restart Your Heart*, Dr. Aseem Desai has thoughtfully laid out a "playbook" full of hope and promise to dispel any and all despair for those dealing with atrial fibrillation. This clear, concise, and comprehensive "game plan for your life" is a holistic approach to living with atrial fibrillation, combining the best of lifestyle guidance and medical science, so you can have a happy, healthy, and successful life. The book's message is about becoming informed and prepared and taking charge of your health.

I can tell you from personal experience that the author of this book truly cares about *you*. Dr. Desai is a man of compassion, courage, and character. He practices *excellence* every day. In this book, there is a game plan for your personal health and performance that will help you improve the quality of your life and face medical challenges as they come. Dr. Desai is a true Hall of Famer who is saving, impacting, and changing lives *every* day, and this book is about to transform your life in a very positive way.

You may not be a football player and have a bronzed bust in Canton, but the playbook Dr. Desai has laid out can give you a Hall of Fame life with a rich legacy of impact on others.

—**David Baker,** President and CEO of
the Pro Football Hall of Fame

Preface

"I was told I had to just live with atrial fibrillation (AFib) and nothing could be done about it." A man in the heart rhythm clinic spoke these words on his one-year anniversary of being in normal sinus rhythm—the normal electrical rhythm of the heart, which starts in an area called the sinus node. It's amazing how a single utterance by someone can spark a fire within you. For me, the spark was this simple statement by an individual who lived with persistent AFib for years. Because his heart was out of rhythm, he felt so poorly he needed to do something more than just "live with it." The journey to his successful outcome was long and arduous, and he wished there had been a simpler way to navigate the process. We smiled at each other when he exited the clinic in normal sinus rhythm, and an idea hit me. People need a straightforward way to deal with this complex disease, and it needs to be presented by experts, who deal with it every day.

I began to search for anything written about AFib. While there were several books that had a lot of useful information and shared moving patient experiences, there was nothing written by an AFib specialist that was a "how to" process of dealing with the condition. As a cardiac electrophysiologist, a physician specializing in heart rhythm disorders, I spend most of my waking hours diagnosing, treating, and monitoring AFib. When I considered the lack of easily accessible information, it seemed only logical that a guide to AFib written by an electrophysiologist was needed.

I've heard . . . time and again . . . people say they were told nothing could be done about their AFib. While it is true that some people with AFib cannot be converted and maintained in a normal rhythm, that number is growing smaller and smaller with advancements in understanding, techniques, and technologies. These advancements have clearly benefited patients with both paroxysmal and persistent AFib. Paroxysmal atrial fibrillation is a type of AFib defined as self-terminating without the need for a medical intervention. Typically, episodes last less than forty-eight hours. Persistent atrial fibrillation is a type of AFib lasting over one week, or which requires a medical intervention, like cardioversion, to terminate. Even for people who live in permanent AFib, there are ways to manage the condition and preserve the quality of life. With any type of AFib, there is the possibility of overcoming it. One needs to define to oneself what overcoming means.

Definition of Overcome (Oxford English Dictionary)

Verb. To succeed in dealing with a problem or difficulty.

Notice that the definition of overcome does not include a statement about victory or cure. To overcome is to deal with a challenge successfully. Well, what defines successfully? If you have AFib, it may mean being in sinus rhythm, which is a normal electrical rhythm in the heart, without recurrence of AFib after ablation. Cardiac ablation is a procedure to scar or destroy tissue in your heart that's allowing incorrect electrical signals to cause an abnormal heart rhythm. This is done with diagnostic catheters that are threaded through blood vessels to your heart where they are used to map your heart's electrical signals.

Or, successfully dealing with the condition could mean a significant reduction in AFib episodes that improves your quality of life because of trigger modification. Or it could mean being in AFib and using medication or a pacemaker to regulate the heartbeat to prevent congestive heart failure and worsening symptoms. And of course, in all cases, it means preventing the most devastating consequence of AFib: stroke.

So when I refer to "overcoming atrial fibrillation," what I am really saying is that you do not have to let this disease define you or your life. You will manage AFib on your terms, not AFib's. *How*, you ask? It's not simple, but it's possible. Living with a health condition is a combination of accepting it, having hope, and having a game plan in dealing with it.

Life is a balance between order and chaos. The heart is no different, both literally and figuratively. Your heart is your body's engine, which normally runs in working order under the authority of its electrical system—amazingly so, if you think about it for a minute. After all, the heart pulses an average of 108,000 beats every day. And when chaos strikes and the heart's electrical system malfunctions, the result is an abnormal rhythm called cardiac arrhythmia.

When it comes to the rhythm of the heart, and the rhythm of life, AFib is the epitome of cardiac chaos. It is the most common cardiac arrhythmia worldwide, and more important, it is a progressive disease. Early detection and early intervention are critical in halting its progression and, in some cases, reversing it. Moreover, it isn't just the heart itself that is the problem when a cardiac arrhythmia appears. AFib has three main consequences: stroke, congestive heart failure, and a range of symptoms affecting quality of life. There is also a growing body of clinical research that indicates that AFib may be associated with an increased risk of dementia.

Writing this book has been illuminating in several ways. First of all, it is clear it is needed. I've spoken with many of my patients and colleagues about the 3-Step guide I developed, and the response has been very positive. Second, I was surprised to hear how many of my patients were told at some point on their health journey, after the diagnosis of AFib was made, that nothing could be done for their AFib. A clear message that came through to me, in doing the research for this book, is that we need more widespread education of the public, health care professionals, and health care systems with regard to the newest treatments for AFib. And, it became clear to me that most people were unaware of the fact that previously "untreatable" patients, those with long-standing persistent AFib, for example, can now have therapeutic options available to them. Lastly, I'll share with you that writing this book for a diverse group of readers was a challenge.

I wanted the material to be relatable and relevant as a practical guide, yet I wanted it to go into more detail for those people who were interested in the science of AFib. One of the biggest challenges has been taking complicated ideas and concepts and translating them into something people can find easy to read and useful. Atul Gawande brings this point forward in his book *The Checklist Manifesto*. He writes, "After a century of incredible discovery most diseases have proved to be far more particular and difficult to treat . . . Medicine has become the art of managing extreme complexity." AFib is all about managing extreme complexity. But we do it every single day.

This book is designed to be a resource for everyone interested in the topic of AFib. That being said, it discusses practical tools that help us all optimize our health and well-being.

The concepts expressed in this book are the result of many, many years of experience in treating patients with AFib. Please keep in mind that other health care professionals may have different views on this subject matter. Finally, to be clear, this book is not a substitute for a professional medical evaluation and treatment plan.

Acknowledgments

I would like to thank Dr. Lindsay Desai, my thoughtful advisor, wife, and best friend, who has stood by me in the epic task of writing a book. Her unwavering belief in me has been the rock upon which I paved my path in this literary journey. She has provided critically important and valuable feedback in developing this book, from cover to cover.

Much gratitude is owed to my entire team at Greenleaf Book Group for their hard work, advice, expertise, and encouragement. This includes Sam Alexander, Stephanie Bouchard, Justin Branch, Erin Brown, Karen Cakebread, Neil Gonzalez, Tyler LeBleu, Olivia McCoy, O'Licia Parker-Smith, Kristine Peyre-Ferry, and countless other people working behind the scenes.

Additional thanks go out to my contributing editors, Nathan Hassall, Rhonda Winchell Sharp, and Patricia Wooster. They provided important developmental/content feedback early in the book writing process.

I would like to thank my talented medical illustrator, Samantha Stutzman. She helped transform my knowledge and ideas into creative expression, all for the sole purpose of helping readers understand the concepts discussed in the book.

And a special expression of gratitude to the women and men I have had the privilege of partnering with to improve their health and well-being.

Finally, I want to express my gratitude to you, the person who picked up this book. Thank you from the bottom of my heart.

Introduction

"Rhythm is sound in motion. It is related to the pulse, the heartbeat, the way we breathe. It rises and falls. It takes us into ourselves; it takes us out of ourselves."

—**Edward Hirsch,** American poet

"Listen to your body and don't brush off health issues that could be career ending, or worse, life ending. AFib was a curveball I didn't see coming."

—**Kenley Jansen,** Major League Baseball pitcher

One Man's Story

On a cold Chicago winter day in 1973, I woke up to a nightmare. I was three years old at the time and I found myself in an unfamiliar bed—in an equally unfamiliar room—completely disoriented. The room was dimly lit, but I could make out the figure of a short, heavyset man at the door. Our next-door neighbor stood in the imposing doorway trying to find the words to explain to a little boy that his dad just had a massive heart attack. Of course, being so young, I had no idea what that meant. But my deep-seated memory recalls feeling intense, unstoppable, earth-shaking fear, and the need to . . . breathe. However, it wasn't my dad's time yet. This thirty-seven-year-old Indian man—husband, father, and physician—would live another day. He was never the same, though. A heart attack can shake the sturdiest of us. From then on, he lived with the constant anxiety of having another heart attack and leaving his family unprotected.

Fast-forward twenty years. I was attending medical school at Northwestern University, as a participant in the Honors Program in Medical Education (HPME). In this program, participants were simultaneously accepted into university and medical school as high school seniors. The purpose of this program was to enable undergraduate, premed students to pursue a liberal arts degree and have a well-rounded education—without the concern of getting into medical school.

At that time, my passion was philosophy. I never would have guessed that the cognitive training required for a philosophy degree would provide me with the deductive and inductive reasoning skills needed to make diagnoses in heart rhythm disorders. When I was a second-year student, I moved from the dorm to an on-campus apartment. On January 5, 1993, around 4 a.m., I received a call from my uncle that my dad died suddenly, while visiting his sister in India. It was the week before my clinical pharmacology final exam, so my brain was memorizing lists of drugs and their interactions. As you can imagine, I had little bandwidth for processing the news about my dad.

After the phone call, the following weeks were a blur. The next thing I knew I was on a transatlantic flight with my brother. We sat in our seats, completely and utterly in shock. I kept asking myself, *Is this really happening?* The flight was long, and when we finally arrived, I found my dad's cold, lifeless body lying in an ambulance, which had transported him from his hometown to Mumbai after he died. I was completely numb. For any of you who have suddenly lost a loved one, you understand the feeling of devastation that irreversibly impacts your life and the life of your family.

A few years later, in 1996, at twenty-five years old, I was in an internal medicine residency at Stanford University Medical Center. During this time, I developed a severe medical illness that would challenge me on many more occasions to come. As I first heard the diagnosis, I took a deep breath, probably the deepest I would ever take. I walked out of the doctor's office in a daze and a fair amount of denial. I often remember this experience when I speak with my patients, because I know they also have the same kind of feelings when they first learn they have a medical problem.

It probably took me a good two weeks before mustering the courage to move forward and try to develop a plan of action. All my previous education was good training and I knew the first thing to do was learn more about the condition—risk factors, causes, and mechanisms. I spent a fair amount of time at bookstores and libraries. The next step was to explore different treatment options.

I knew I had to find a health care professional with extensive expertise in evaluating and managing this medical problem.

At the time there were not many doctor-review websites, as the Internet was still in its earliest phase. So, I made my decision based on talking with several physicians who knew colleagues in the area of expertise I needed. I researched the qualifications, education, and experience of the providers on the list I'd constructed. Beyond being "good on paper," there were certain key personality and behavioral traits I felt were necessary: being a mindful listener, being clear and concise when speaking to make visits efficient and productive, being confident in their knowledge and experience yet willing to admit limitations and ask for help from colleagues or academic medical centers, and being encouraging and supportive in the treatment process.

I suffered several exacerbations of this medical problem as I continued my professional training. This was difficult for both myself and my family, who took it pretty hard. With each of these exacerbations, I learned something new about handling and controlling the disease and how I responded to it. These experiences became a compendium of behaviors, which I could "go to" when knocked down. This resulted in the idea of a resilience toolbox that I have drawn upon to this day. From the start, I knew I needed to be an advocate for my own health and also build a support network to rely on during the really challenging times.

Time kept marching on, as it always does, until June 2018, when my world—once again—came to a screeching halt. In the quiet morning hours of a California June day, my cell phone blared its ringtone throughout the house, nearly waking up our two-year-old son. It was a nurse at a Chicago-area hospital telling me my mom was admitted, twenty-four hours prior, for shortness of breath. The admittance was for "observation" but took a turn for the worse very quickly. As the nurse was trying to relay what had happened to bring her to the hospital, I heard in the background loud beeping sounds and a chorus of people shouting at the same time. The sounds immediately triggered my thoughts to race and my breath became shallow. Those sounds are never good sounds to hear in a hospital.

Most of you have never witnessed a hospital code, although you may have seen one acted out on television. Medical television shows use codes to heighten tension and drama. And a hospital code is dramatic because what is happening is dramatic. A code is issued when, for instance, someone is experiencing a cardiopulmonary arrest. This dreaded event commonly occurs when the lungs shut down, the heart shuts down, or most often both shut down. A cardiopulmonary arrest can be due to several different causes.

A code is complete chaos. A human being is dying on the bed and people are doing their best to save the person. You can imagine how the adrenaline pumping in the collective group of doctors, nurses, pharmacists, and respiratory therapists mirrors the IV adrenaline that is being pumped into a patient's veins to maintain blood flow to the brain.

I asked the nurse, "Are you coding my mom?" There was a brief pause, then a word no one would want to hear in this situation: "Yes."

I couldn't believe what was happening. No one in our family had any idea she was in the hospital. In some ways, I wasn't surprised how we found out, though. It was very much like my mom to keep her health issues to herself for fear of burdening her family. That being said, finding out like this was one of the greatest burdens I would ever bear. Thankfully, my wife was right next to me when the call came, and in her amazingly calm and level-headed way, she made arrangements for me to travel from California to Chicago.

In what seemed like a flash, I grabbed a few belongings, flew from Orange County's John Wayne Airport to Chicago's O'Hare, hopped in a cab to the hospital, and walked quickly into the intensive care unit. As I rushed into my mom's room, I saw her lying motionless on the bed. A tube down her throat and intravenous medications were the only things keeping her alive. She felt very cold. There was a striking similarity to the way I had seen my dad years ago.

She was almost gone, and from my medical training, I knew the likelihood of her recovering was next to nothing. And if she did live, it would have been a terrible life for her, and certainly not what she would have wanted. Shortly after, I found myself withdrawing life support. I sat there and held her hand as I watched the respiratory therapist remove the endotracheal tube. Then I watched the heart rhythm go from fast, to slow, to flatline. My mom was one of the healthiest people I knew. We had spoken on the phone only a few days prior. She was getting ready to visit us and spend some quality time with her grandchildren. But now that wasn't going to happen.

Something that really hit home with me about this experience was this: *Always* keep your loved ones informed of your health.

You may think you don't want to burden them, but trust me, finding out when it's too late for them to help you is a far greater burden to carry.

As I look back on these experiences, I have a greater understanding of their remarkably transformative effect on me. My father's passing was my catalyst to becoming a healer. My medical condition was the catalyst for understanding what it's like to live with a chronic disease. My mother's passing was the catalyst for knowing what it feels like to let go of someone's life when that someone is the same someone who gave you yours. I suppose, in many ways, these cumulative experiences have served as the catalyst for authoring this book.

My hope, in writing this book about AFib for you, is to connect with you through these pages. It's for all of us to find common ground—patients, allied health professionals, health administrators, and doctors. As you will learn in the pages that follow, AFib is that common ground. It can happen to any of us. This cardiac chaos does not discriminate. This cardiac chaos is strong. *But the human spirit is stronger.*

Anyone's Story

There are many people who are living with AFib, which is due to several different causes, many of which are clear. However, for others, there is no obvious cause. I've seen patients as young as eighteen and as old as one hundred. Regardless of the cause, the treatment course is often first influenced by age, overall health, and a person's goals. The disease can afflict any of us when we reach a certain age. Each person with AFib has their own unique set of circumstances, which leads to the first AFib event.

It is worth restating this point: Each person with AFib has a unique set of symptoms and circumstances that lead to the first event. In electrophysiology (EP) we call this "the perfect storm." It may help to answer the question most people will have when they learn they have AFib: "Why did I go into AFib now?" To answer this question, we'll review the stories of four different people from different walks of life, who were faced with that first moment of AFib—and didn't know what their physical symptoms meant or indicated about their health. That's a very common thread. It is why we consider AFib an "electrical cancer."

These are their four stories.

Chris is an eighteen-year-old, healthy college student, though with a family history of cardiac arrhythmias. One day he experienced sudden unbearable heart racing and dizziness. He couldn't breathe. It terrified him and his family.

Kelsey is a forty-year-old, successful real estate agent without any history of heart disease. However, one day she experienced profound and unexplainable fatigue. Subsequently, she would have these "waves" of fatigue—some days she would feel great and other days terrible. Depression got the better of her, and she withdrew from life. She felt her breath fade.

Tom is a sixty-year-old physician with a history of high blood pressure. He is also an avid runner. Tom has helped many people improve their health. Yet one day, he found himself on the other side of the equation, as a patient being rushed to the emergency room.

His breathing became shallow on the ambulance ride over, and his head was spinning with thoughts of what was going to happen.

Pat is an eighty-nine-year-old retired schoolteacher who volunteers at a nearby hospital. She has a history of diabetes, sleep apnea, and coronary artery bypass surgery. She experienced chronic general malaise that she attributed to getting older. It was almost as if she couldn't take a deep breath. Like something was restricting her.

What do all of these people have in common? Atrial fibrillation. The electrical epidemic. Arthritis of the electrical system. Electrical cancer. We use a lot of analogies to describe the significance and impact of this disease on our planet. It is more widespread than we think. One of the biggest challenges is that the disease varies from individual to individual, which makes it complicated to treat.

We will describe the different ways that Chris, Kelsey, Tom, and Pat each overcame AFib in the Case Studies section at the end of this book.

Book Overview

This book outlines three steps for managing AFib: **(1) Be Informed**, **(2) Be Prepared**, and **(3) Be in Control**. Each of these is a unit divided into three chapters. At the end of most of the chapters are **Action Items** that represent practical steps you can take toward overcoming AFib. Keep in mind that overcoming it may mean something different to each person. A synopsis of each chapter is given below, for quick referencing.

Step 1: Be Informed

It is important to note that the chapters in this section are fairly technical and read similar to a textbook. Chapter 1, Cause, discusses the "what and why" of AFib—what it is, why it happens, and what to do when you are diagnosed. A key point is to identify and manage risk factors and triggers for AFib. In Chapter 2, Confirmation, you'll find diagnostic tools, tests, and questions to ask an AFib specialist. Chapter 3, Control, includes treatments such as drugs, devices, ablation, and combinations of different therapies. It also includes frequently asked questions, because the answers to these questions can help you and your provider make informed decisions about treatments.

Step 2: Be Prepared

This section focuses on dealing with the diagnosis and condition on mental and emotional levels, which is just as important as the physical level (see Chapter 4). Chapter 5, Build a Toolbox, actually applies to any medical diagnosis. It discusses practical methods one can employ to maintain quality of life even in the presence of the condition. And Chapter 6 outlines how to enlist health care professionals and social support networks to help navigate the health care system and stay strong.

Step 3: Be in Control

Chapter 7 is about monitoring the disease to prevent progression, and here we discuss newer technologies to track heart rhythm disorders. For some reputable informational sources, see Chapter 8. And Chapter 9 focuses on how combining all the steps leads to taking charge of your overall health, not just AFib.

Finally, the Case Studies section is a critical one to review, because it shows you that you are not alone with AFib. This is one of the most important sections to read, because the many ways in which people dealt with their AFib may apply to your circumstances, and, more important, may help you.

Now that you have a map of the book, let's begin.

STEP 1

BE INFORMED

CHAPTER 1

Cause

"The improvement of understanding is for two ends: first, our own increase of knowledge; secondly, to enable us to deliver that knowledge to others."

—**John Locke,** English philosopher and physician

"I knew there was always something funny about my heart . . . I got a little scared, because it [AFib] didn't seem like it was going away."

—**Larry Bird,** former professional basketball player, coach, and team executive

Don't Hold Your Breath

Eric is forty-five and overweight. He had paroxysmal atrial fibrillation, which failed to respond to sotalol, an antiarrhythmic drug used to suppress AFib. He was scheduled for an ablation. At a pre-op visit, his wife mentioned he snored regularly. When I asked Eric how his sleep was, he said he thought it was "fine," but that he always felt tired in the morning when he woke up. Upon hearing this history, I ordered an in-office sleep study that found Eric had severe obstructive sleep apnea. He was started on continuous positive airway pressure (CPAP) therapy, which is a machine that delivers pressurized air to keep the airways open.

Eric had an implantable monitor in place, so we could track his AFib easily. Within a week of starting CPAP, his AFib episodes literally resolved. We subsequently canceled the ablation procedure and after six months of instituting CPAP, no further AFib has been documented on the implantable monitor. Eric now feels rested when he wakes up in the morning. And good sleep hygiene has altered his overall sense of well-being for the better. Improving his sleep has resulted in a positive upward spiral that has improved his personal and work relationships, productivity, and life satisfaction. Because of improved sleep, he now has more energy to exercise. Regular exercise steered him toward a better diet. The positive spiral resulted in a weight loss of thirty pounds over three months. All of this without a drug or an ablation. Just treating an AFib trigger. In Eric's case, sleep apnea was the trigger.

The Basics of the Heart's Electrical System

A general premise for why atrial fibrillation occurs is that it represents the perfect storm of nature meeting nurture. In this case, the nature indicator would be any genetic predisposition to electrical abnormalities. The nurture side would be AFib risk factors and

Blood Flow in the Heart

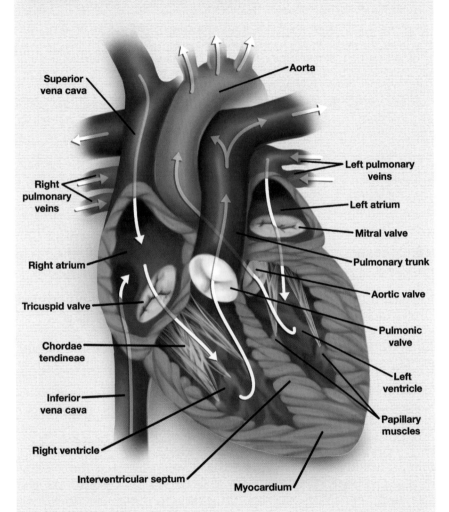

Deoxygenated blood enters the right atrium via the superior
and inferior vena cavae (veins), enters the right ventricle
through the tricuspid valve, and exits the right ventricle to the
lungs through the pulmonic valve. Blood receives fresh oxygen
then enters the left atrium via the pulmonary veins, enters the
left ventricle through the mitral valve, and exits the left ventricle
to the rest of the body through the aortic valve.

Figure 1

triggers due to associated medical conditions and lifestyle influ-
ences, as described later in this chapter.

The first step in dealing with atrial fibrillation is to understand
what it is. But before that, let's go over the heart and its different
components.

Your heart is an engine, which has three basic components: a set
of electrical pathways that power it (cardiac conduction system),
a plumbing system that feeds it oxygen-rich blood (left and right
coronary arteries), and a set of four valves that keep blood moving in
one direction (tricuspid, pulmonic, mitral, and aortic valves).

The cardiac conduction system starts in an area called the
sinoatrial (SA) node. The SA node, commonly called the sinus
node, is a group of cells at the top part of the right atrium, which
sets the heartbeat. These cells are influenced by states of adrenaline in the body. Here, the brain and the heart interface via
the autonomic nervous system (ANS) to produce impulses that
move through the heart, which cause the muscle fibers to contract. The ANS is the branch of the nervous system that controls
all basic bodily functions including the heartbeat, breathing, and
the gastrointestinal system.

There are pathways that connect the sinus node to the atrioventricular (AV) node. This is a group of cells in the center of the
electrical system. They act as a "tollbooth," controlling impulses
from going too fast, as they travel from the top to the bottom
(atria to ventricles) of the heart. Continuing with this tollbooth
analogy, the AV node controls the number of "cars" passing
through so that "traffic" doesn't get too backed up and slows
down (called bradycardia) or moves too fast (called tachycardia).

Cardiac Conduction System

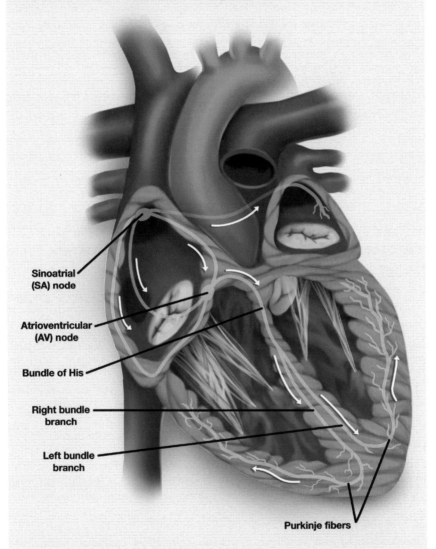

Sinoatrial (SA) node

Atrioventricular (AV) node

Bundle of His

Right bundle branch

Left bundle branch

Purkinje fibers

The heartbeat begins in the sinus node and moves through right and left atria via specialized fibers and an interatrial tract called Bachmann's bundle. The electrical impulse then moves through the AV node and exits to the right and left ventricles via the bundle branches. The bundle branches rapidly activate muscular contraction of the ventricles.

Figure 2

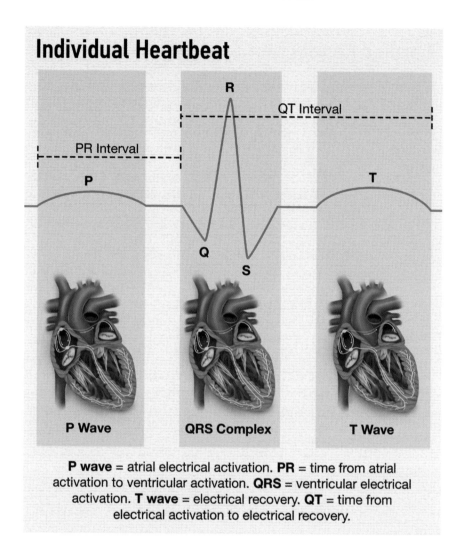

Individual Heartbeat

P wave = atrial electrical activation. PR = time from atrial activation to ventricular activation. QRS = ventricular electrical activation. T wave = electrical recovery. QT = time from electrical activation to electrical recovery.

Figure 3

The electrical pathways then split into the right bundle branch, which causes the right ventricle to contract, and then into the left bundle branch, which causes the left ventricle to contract. After the heart performs its coordinated contraction, and then relaxes the muscle fibers, one complete heartbeat has occurred.

A diagnostic test called an electrocardiogram (EKG) measures the flow of electricity through the heart. An individual heartbeat on the EKG is composed of three sections: a P wave, a QRS complex, and a T wave. These correspond to three distinct events. The P wave is the electrical activation of the right and left atria, the QRS is the electrical activation of the right and left ventricles, and the T wave is the electrical recovery of the ventricles before the next heartbeat. An interval called the PR interval represents the time it takes for an electrical impulse to travel from the sinus node to the AV node. The QT interval is the recovery time of the ventricles. The hallmark sign of atrial fibrillation is the loss of the P wave.

In addition to the normal cardiac conduction system described above, the unique thing about the heart's electrical system is that any of its muscular cells, called cardiomyocytes, can initiate and transmit electrical impulses from any of the four chambers—right atrium, left atrium, right ventricle, and left ventricle. These impulses are caused by the movement of positively and negatively charged ions including sodium, potassium, calcium, and magnesium through proteins called ion channel receptors. To understand this better, let's use the analogy of people living in a house with multiple rooms and doorways connected to each other. The people are the ions, the house is the heart, the rooms are the cells, and the doorways are the ion channel receptors. Just as people move in and out of the rooms through doorways, the ions move in and out of the cell through ion channel receptors. The movement is driven by electrical gradients.

These gradients occur when there is a relative difference in

Heartbeat's Effect on the Ion Channel Receptors

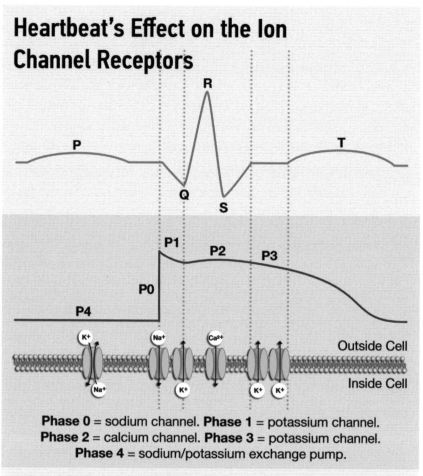

Phase 0 = sodium channel. Phase 1 = potassium channel.
Phase 2 = calcium channel. Phase 3 = potassium channel.
Phase 4 = sodium/potassium exchange pump.

Ion Channel Receptors Analogy

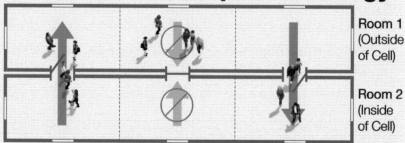

This figure demonstrates the following from top to bottom: A single heartbeat on an EKG, a cardiac action potential (individual heart cell) and ion channel opening/closing sequence, and an analogy of ions and channels to people in rooms of a house.

Figures 4 and 5

concentration inside and outside the cells of these different ions. When an individual heartbeat starts, the sodium channel ion receptor opens because there's more sodium outside the cell than inside. Once the doorway opens, the room (the cell) is flooded. When the number of ions hits a certain threshold, the door shuts and another one opens. This causes a domino effect, which drives the electrical impulse.

Mechanisms of Cardiac Arrhythmias

What happens when the aforementioned process goes wrong?

Cardiac arrhythmias happen, of which atrial fibrillation is the most common type. There are benign ones, such as premature beats and supraventricular tachycardia, and malignant ones, such as ventricular tachycardia and fibrillation, and ones in between, such as atrial fibrillation. Cardiac arrhythmias occur due to three basic mechanisms: reentry, triggered activity, and automaticity. Arrhythmias can be the result of one of these mechanisms or a combination of them. The cellular basis for these is a result of the ion channels described above. In fact, the drugs that treat arrhythmias work by modifying these ion channels. Remember the doorway analogy above? Well, drugs can block a doorway. And this affects the way an electrical impulse is generated and moves and whether it is allowed through the doorway or blocked from entering.

Reentry occurs when an electrical impulse gets caught in a vicious circular loop that causes the heart to beat rapidly. Some of the best examples of reentry include supraventricular tachycardia, Wolff-Parkinson-White syndrome, atrial flutter, and ventricular tachycardia due to scar tissue, which may be present if you've experienced a prior heart attack, for example.

Imagine a merry-go-round at an amusement park. As the ride spins in a circle, you can jump on and off. If it goes too fast, you can't jump off. That is reentry. Treating reentry is possible with medication that slows the merry-go-round or ablation that stops the merry-go-round. In many cases, the latter is preferred. Another way to think about reentry is like a runner on a race-track. The runner is the abnormal heart rhythm that is caught in a vicious circular loop. Medication for reentrant arrhythmias is like putting a series of hurdles on the racetrack to slow down the runner. Doing an ablation is like building a wall on the racetrack to stop the runner.

Triggered activity is when electrical cells build up with cal-cium ions, which can generate an abnormal heartbeat. This is not related to the dietary intake of calcium. It is related to the inabil-ity of the cell to maintain proper calcium ion balance inside and outside of it. The hallmark of triggered activity is that fast heart rates cause more calcium to accumulate, and that increases the likelihood of an arrhythmia. A good example of this phenomenon is a rhythm called idiopathic ventricular tachycardia. Here, people often experience it during exercise when the heart rate is fast. It is caused by a group of abnormal cells in either the right or left ventricle. Because triggered activity is dependent on a calcium ion mechanism, a calcium channel blocker drug is often used to treat arrhythmias related to triggered activity.

Automaticity occurs when abnormal cells with spontaneous electrical activity fire. This means that there are cells that have the ability to create their own beat, independent of the normal heartbeat. Often, arrhythmias related to abnormal automaticity get triggered under states of elevated adrenaline. Adrenaline is a

Arrhythmia Mechanisms

Mechanisms of arrhythmias as seen on cardiac action potential

Reentry - electrical impulse gets caught in a vicious circular loop that causes the heart to beat rapidly

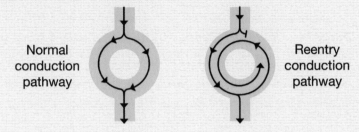

Triggered activity - electrical cells build up with calcium ions that can generate an abnormal heartbeat

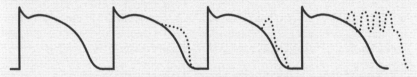

Automaticity - abnormal cells with spontaneous electrical activity fire

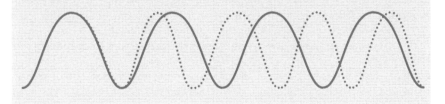

Figure 6a

substance your body produces under stress or when physically active. Because stress can be a trigger, examples of arrhythmias that use the automaticity mechanism include premature atrial or premature ventricular contractions, automatic atrial tachycardia, and automatic ventricular tachycardia.

Round and Around the Merry-Go-Round: A Case of Reentry

CASE STUDY: BRENDA

Brenda is a sixty-one-year-old volunteer at a soup kitchen, who has dedicated much of her life to the service of others. For her last birthday, her son bought her a new Apple Watch Series 4 with the EKG feature (Apple's ECG app). She loved how it tracked her physical activity and gave her a "nudge" when she was behind on her daily steps goal. However, she began noticing periods of time when her heartbeat would suddenly increase to 150 beats per minute, even when at rest. During these times, which could last up to several hours, she felt intense fatigue and dizziness. These events would sometimes occur at the most inopportune times—when she was hosting a dinner party, when she was out shopping for weekly groceries, or when she was volunteering at the soup kitchen.

She finally caught one of these events on the Apple Watch ECG and showed it to her doctor, who diagnosed her with a rhythm called atrial flutter. Her diagnostic workup revealed some right atrial enlargement on the echocardiogram but otherwise was unremarkable. Since there was no identifiable cause for the atrial flutter and it was recurrent, she was faced with a decision to take a lifelong medication or consider a catheter ablation procedure. Brenda's resting heart rate was in the 50-beats-per-minute range, so taking any cardiac medication for her rhythm was likely to drop it even further and cause significant side effects.

She underwent an atrial flutter ablation procedure. Here, the diagnosis was what is called typical right atrial cavo-tricuspid isthmus dependent flutter. This arrhythmia is the hallmark of a reentry mechanism. There is an area of slower electrical movement in the tissue located between the tricuspid valve and the inferior vena cava vein in the right atrium. The circuit typically moves about 300 beats per minute around the right atrium like a merry-go-round that doesn't stop. The AV node protects the ventricles from going 300 beats per minute by blocking every other impulse from the atrium. Therefore, the typical pulse rate in atrial flutter is about 150 beats per minute (half of 300).

The hallmark of atrial flutter is that it is often very regular, as opposed to atrial fibrillation, which is usually irregular. Atrial flutter is commonly associated with atrial fibrillation, and up to 30 percent of people who have isolated atrial flutter will go on to develop atrial fibrillation at some point later in life. For this reason, electrophysiologists are very aggressive about stopping atrial flutter. Fortunately, the success rate of atrial flutter ablation is upwards of 90 percent with very low risk, since the rhythm is on the right side of the heart. Brenda underwent the ablation successfully and has not had any other rhythm problems. It took sixty minutes to do the procedure and she went home the same day. She truly feels like she has her life back. And everyone at the soup kitchen is happier for it.

Okay, enough about the basic science of cardiac electrophysiology. Now it's time to turn to the crux of the book, atrial fibrillation.

Types of Atrial Fibrillation

The unique thing about atrial fibrillation is that it can involve all three mechanisms of arrhythmias: reentry, triggered activity, and automaticity.

To analogize this, imagine a series of broken wires in your home. These wires have a break in the insulation that can send off

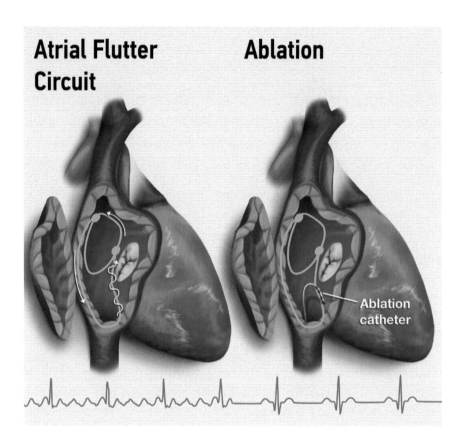

Atrial Flutter Circuit

Ablation

Ablation catheter

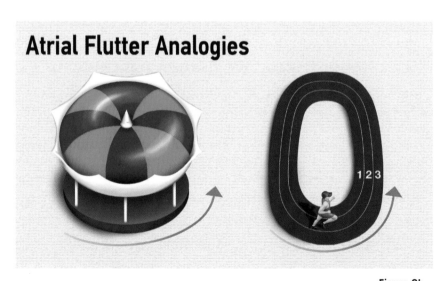

Atrial Flutter Analogies

1 2 3

sparks of electricity. When the sparks occur frequently enough, or for a long enough period of time, they can start a fire. In the heart, the broken wires are abnormal cells located in anatomic structures capable of independent electrical activity (automaticity). These anatomic structures most commonly include the pulmonary veins (PV foci), but also may include other sites such as the superior vena cava, ligament of Marshall, left atrial appendage, coronary sinus, and posterior wall (non-PV foci).

There are four types of atrial fibrillation: paroxysmal, persistent, long-standing persistent, and permanent. Picture AFib as fire: It can come and go (paroxysmal), or it can burn continuously (persistent). In fact, drugs act like duct tape around the wires' insulation breaks, and ablation is like repairing the insulation, in many but not all cases.

When atrial fibrillation begins (paroxysmal), it starts with the abnormal cells mentioned above, most commonly cells in the pulmonary veins. These cells act as triggers. They create premature atrial contractions, often referred to as "skipped beats," "extra beats," or "flutters." Now, premature beats are common benign causes of palpitation symptoms in the majority of people. However, if a patient is at risk for AFib and has a sufficient number of premature beats, these can act as major starters of the fire. In other cases, the abnormal cells can be drivers of the arrhythmia (rapid activity sustaining atrial fibrillation). In some cases, atrial fibrillation can result from other abnormal rhythms. A good example is Wolff-Parkinson-White syndrome. With this condition, an additional electrical connection, an accessory pathway, causes rapid heart rates (supraventricular tachycardia) that can trigger atrial fibrillation.

As atrial fibrillation progresses, with more frequent and

longer-lasting episodes, more circuits are created, and it becomes a vicious cycle. This is where the phrase "AFib begets AFib" comes from. As AFib progresses, soon large sections of atrial anatomy may contain abnormal scar tissue that facilitates sustaining atrial fibrillation. If atrial fibrillation occurs for more than seven days in a row, it is called persistent. If it occurs for more than a year continuously, it is called long-standing persistent.

These are all descriptions of mechanisms of AFib. Permanent AFib, though, is not really a mechanism; it is a decision a doctor and patient make together. Here, the decision is made to leave the heart in atrial fibrillation because any additional attempts to maintain sinus rhythm are likely to have greater risk than benefit.

If you want to use a different analogy, AFib can be thought of as electrical cancer. Initially, the tumor is limited (paroxysmal, pulmonary veins). As AFib continues, more cells are produced to the point of metastatic electrical cancer. It can still be treated, but may require more than one modality, similar to real cancer. Sometimes, with advanced cancer, you may need surgery and chemotherapy or surgery and radiation therapy. Sometimes you need surgery, chemo, and radiation. In the same way with AFib, sometimes you need a combination of treatments to overcome the arrhythmia: ablation and a drug, or ablation and a pacemaker. Sometimes, you need an ablation, a drug, and a pacemaker. The correct combination will be determined by your physician and health care providers.

There are methods to diagnose where the broken wires are (rhythm monitors, electrophysiology study) and manage the insulation breaks (meds = duct tape, ablation = sealing the insulation).

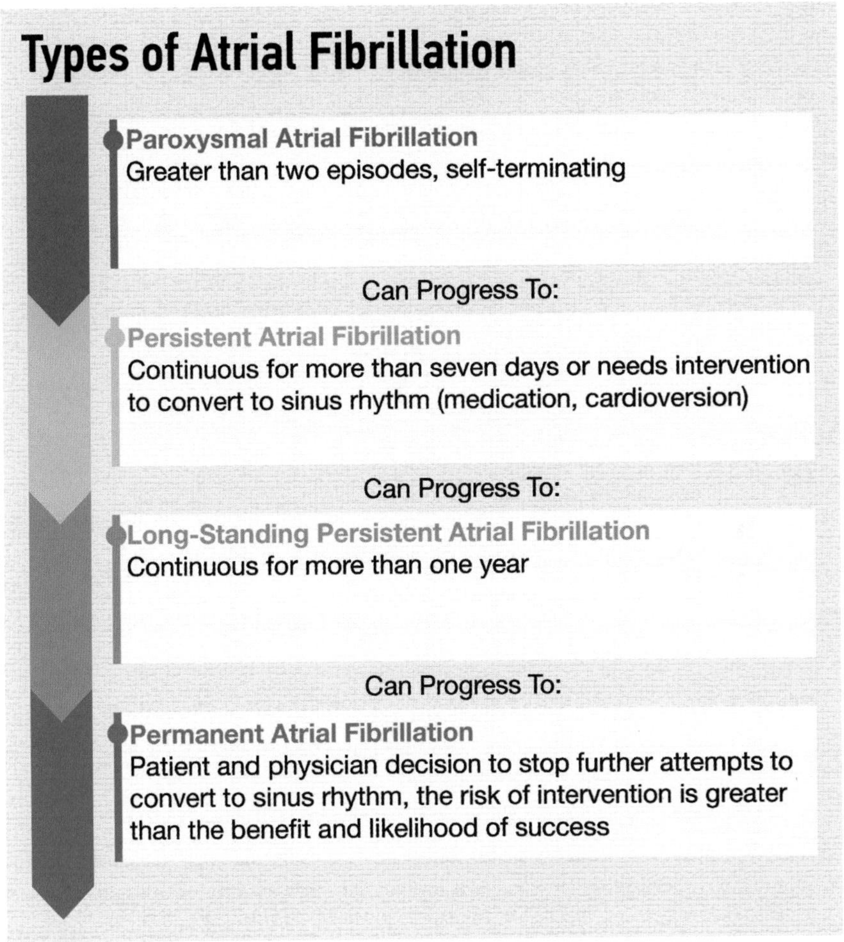

Types of Atrial Fibrillation

◆Paroxysmal Atrial Fibrillation
Greater than two episodes, self-terminating

Can Progress To:

◆Persistent Atrial Fibrillation
Continuous for more than seven days or needs intervention
to convert to sinus rhythm (medication, cardioversion)

Can Progress To:

◆Long-Standing Persistent Atrial Fibrillation
Continuous for more than one year

Can Progress To:

◆Permanent Atrial Fibrillation
Patient and physician decision to stop further attempts to
convert to sinus rhythm, the risk of intervention is greater
than the benefit and likelihood of success

Figure 7a

We will come back to this analogy later. The ultimate outcome
with atrial fibrillation can include stroke, because blood coagulates
when it does not move properly; congestive heart failure, because
the heart muscle weakens due to rapid irregular activity; and various symptoms, which can range from palpitations to generalmal-
aise and fatigue.

Risk Factors for Atrial Fibrillation

There are several risk factors for atrial fibrillation. These include being over age sixty-five, obesity, high blood pressure, diabetes, thyroid disease, sleep apnea, heavy alcohol use, coronary artery disease, valvular heart disease, and advanced lung disease. We discuss some of these in more detail below. In general, as you can see, poor health is a risk factor for AFib.

Genetic AFib does exist—we tend to see it in patients who are very young, often with a family history of AFib at young ages. In the past, we would refer to patients without structural heart disease as having "lone atrial fibrillation" but this term is no longer used in the field of electrophysiology (EP). It is now suspected that patients without structural heart disease develop atrial fibrillation as a result of genetic and environmental factors. In other words, a combination of nature and nurture.

Age Over Sixty-Five

Aging is a key contributor to AFib. It's like arthritis of the electrical system. Just as scar tissue can form in your knee, shoulder, or hip joint, similar scar tissue can form between healthy electrical tissue and form the substrate for arrhythmias. The prevalence of AFib in the adult population doubles with each advancing decade of age, from 0.5 percent at ages fifty to fifty-nine to 9 percent at ages eighty to eighty-nine.

The risk of stroke in the setting of AFib similarly increases with age, being highest in people over the age of seventy-five. This was shown quite elegantly in the Framingham Heart Study,

Prevalence of Atrial Fibrillation by Decade of Age: Framingham Study

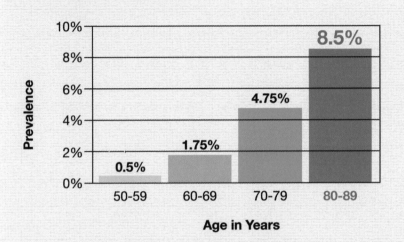

Projected Number of Patients with Atrial Fibrillation by 2050

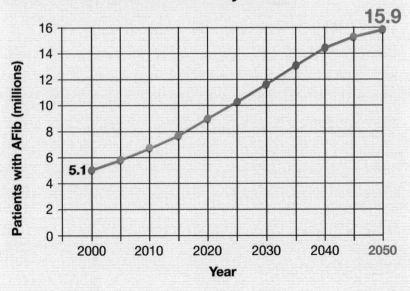

Figure 7b

one of the largest cardiovascular longitudinal cohort studies in the world. It began in 1948 with 5,209 adult subjects from Framingham, Massachusetts, and it is currently on its third generation of participants. This study is where most of our current knowledge about the risk factors of heart disease is derived. It is also where our understanding of the effects of diet and exercise on the heart has originated. The study is a project of the National Heart, Lung, and Blood Institute in collaboration with Boston University.

Furthermore, since our world's population is living longer due to advancements in disease prevention and treatment, the projected number of people with AFib in the future is staggering. In fact, it is estimated that in the United States alone by the year 2050, 16 million people will have AFib.

Obesity

Obesity is another risk factor for AFib. In part, this is because it can cause associated medical problems such as diabetes and high blood pressure, which contribute to developing the arrhythmia, and in part because obesity itself can stress the body and heart. Increased body fat is also associated with increased fat around the heart (epicardial fat), which can contribute to AFib. This increase in epicardial fat can sometimes make it more difficult to get an ablation lesion (known as a transmural lesion) all the way through the heart's electrical tissue. Some ablation studies have shown that patients with obesity who achieve significant weight loss before AFib ablation have a lower rate of recurrent AFib post-ablation compared to similar patients who have not lost weight. This underscores the fact that AFib is a manifestation of a systemic disease. Thus, a keen area of focus in the ablation world is risk-factor modification before and after ablation.

High Blood Pressure

High blood pressure is both a risk factor and a trigger for AFib. Long-standing and uncontrolled high blood pressure increases the pressure in the left atrium, causing enlargement (dilatation), which can lead to AFib. An acute increase in blood pressure (a salty meal, missing med doses) can act as a trigger for an AFib episode. Similar to the other risk factors, managing high blood pressure is critical in the management of AFib. Modifying diet, by reducing salt, caffeine, and alcohol, and exercising regularly are two great ways to lower blood pressure. You've probably heard that "prescription" before, but correcting diet and adding exercise works so well that it's worth noting again and again.

Magnesium supplementation can also help. Fortunately, some of the drugs used for blood pressure also help with AFib. These are beta-blockers and calcium channel blockers. Beta-blockers are essentially adrenaline modifiers, which reduce the frequency of premature beats that can trigger AFib, control the heart rate during AFib, and help control blood pressure. These include metoprolol, atenolol, carvedilol, propranolol, and nebivolol, to name a few. As for the calcium channel blockers, there are two types: dihydropyridine and nondihydropyridine. Amlodipine is an example of a dihydropyridine, but it is not used for atrial fibrillation because it has no significant impact on the electrical system. Verapamil and diltiazem are examples of nondihydropyridine, and they can help control the heart rate in atrial fibrillation, as well as reduce the frequency of premature beats, which trigger AFib.

Sleep Apnea

Remember the term "lone atrial fibrillation" mentioned earlier? It is now increasingly recognized that undiagnosed sleep apnea may be the cause in many cases.

Physicians have a low threshold for recommending a sleep apnea evaluation because it is strongly connected to AFib. Sleep apnea is a condition where a person stops breathing while sleeping, either as a result of airway obstruction (obstructive sleep apnea, or OSA) or the brain's control of sleep (central sleep apnea). Obstructive sleep apnea can either occur as a result of obesity (for example, a larger neck results in more pressure on the airway) or if the person has anatomical abnormalities with the chin or jaw. In the case of central sleep apnea, the brain doesn't send signals properly to the muscles that control breathing. It is therefore important to note that you can have sleep apnea without being overweight or snoring.

Often, people do not realize they have sleep apnea because they cannot recall it. The mind has an amnesic quality during sleep. This is why something may happen in the middle of the night but you don't have recollection of it the next day. Furthermore, if you suffer from sleep apnea, your partner may not know it if he or she is a sound sleeper. The most common symptoms and signs of sleep apnea are daytime sleepiness, fatigue, and snoring. As a result of either obstructive or central sleep apnea, repetitive drops in oxygen can stress the heart. Furthermore, sleep apnea is associated with an increased risk of traffic accidents and work injuries.

People with sleep apnea do not necessarily have AFib while they have apnea events. This is a noteworthy point because many people say to me, "Sleep apnea can't be causing my AFib because I don't get AFib in the middle of the night." But at least two of the suspected mechanisms for sleep apnea are associated with AFib: (1) repetitive drops in oxygen can cause changes in the atria, which facilitate the development of AFib, and (2) repetitive drops in oxygen stimulate the production of adrenaline, which can trigger AFib.

Low levels of oxygen, called hypoxia, shorten an electrical property of the heart called the atrial refractory period. The atrial refractory period refers to the time it takes for a cell in the atrium to recover before it can produce or transmit another electrical impulse. When the atrial refractory period shortens, more premature beats can occur in a shorter period of time, which increases the chances of triggering AFib.

Screening for sleep apnea can occur with a home study. If it is abnormal, or if the suspicion is high that the patient has sleep apnea because there have been witnessed apneic events, then a formal in-office sleep study can be done. In this case, CPAP therapy uses a machine to deliver air and oxygen to open the airways.

When people hear the words "sleep study" and "sleep apnea," often what is immediately conjured up is a large contraption that forces air into you and negatively impacts your sleep. These impressions are frequently a result of an improperly fitting mask, suboptimal CPAP programming, or insufficient education about the tools and technologies. Other ways to treat sleep apnea include dental appliances that move the jaw and reduce tongue obstruction of the airway, and surgery (like removing large tonsils/adenoids that may be contributing to obstruction). There are even implantable devices that stimulate nerves involved with the tongue to help move it out of the way. In short, when it comes to sleep apnea, have a low threshold for evaluation if you have unexplained AFib.

CASE STUDY: MITCH

I was recently humbled by the case of Mitch, a forty-five-year-old man, who had experienced long-standing persistent AFib for five years. He initially presented with congestive heart failure due to rapid AFib that had been occurring for years without him realizing it. His only symptoms were fatigue and malaise, which he attributed to working too hard. This is a common story. Mitch underwent cardioversions, ablations, drug therapy, and a combination of treatments.

Finally, one day his wife came to his appointment and mentioned in passing that he slept poorly and asked if it may be due to his snoring and periods of not breathing that she'd witnessed. We subsequently did a sleep study and diagnosed him with obstructive sleep apnea. Once treatment was instituted and he was cardioverted again, he remained in sinus rhythm. This is an extreme example of the importance of treating comorbidities associated with AFib to maintain sinus rhythm. One can keep ablating tissue and adding medication, but if the triggers and contributors to AFib are not addressed, the disease will either persist or recur.

The bottom line with AFib is that it does not matter how you get to sinus rhythm (meds, ablation, device, combination); the treatment is *being in* sinus rhythm. Just as AFib begets AFib, sinus rhythm begets sinus rhythm. *The heart is a muscle and being in AFib creates a muscle memory that makes the heart want to stay in AFib.* We just need to change the default muscle memory to that of sinus rhythm. And the longer the heart remains in sinus, the lower the chances of recurrent AFib. A favorite saying I tell my patients is: "Every day of sinus rhythm is a good day and one to celebrate—don't look too far into the future."

Diabetes

Diabetes is considered an independent risk factor for stroke in the setting of AFib. Diabetes causes "microvascular disease" in all the major arterial systems: brain, heart, and peripheral arteries. It is thought that this effect on blood flow to the atria may be, in part, responsible for the contribution of diabetes to AFib. Tight control of blood sugar can lessen the chances of developing AFib and triggering AFib episodes. Furthermore, diabetes often results from obesity, and obesity is a risk factor for AFib as well.

Coronary Artery Disease

Coronary artery disease (CAD), or atherosclerosis of the coronary arteries due to lipid deposition, is a risk factor for AFib. If blood flow is affected within the arteries that feed the atria blood, the result can be scarring of the atria. The scarring can contribute to the development of AFib. A prior heart attack also causes scarring. Oftentimes, patients are on beta-blockers for CAD to prevent heart attacks and improve coronary blood flow. These drugs can also help AFib, which provides a two-for-one benefit to the patient.

Congestive Heart Failure

Congestive heart failure (CHF) can be a significant risk factor for developing AFib, and a temporary worsening of congestive heart failure can trigger an individual AFib episode. There are two types of CHF: systolic and diastolic. Systolic CHF refers to a heart muscle that is weakened and cannot pump effectively, thereby causing backup of fluid throughout the body—most notably in the lungs, extremities, and abdomen. Diastolic CHF is due to a stiff and noncompliant heart that cannot fill with blood properly, which in turn limits how much blood is pumped in a specific cardiac cycle. In both of these conditions, a long-standing overload of fluid results in enlargement and abnormal functioning of the atrial chambers. CHF and AFib have a reciprocal relationship. CHF can trigger AFib and AFib can trigger CHF. The latter occurs when the heart rate runs fast and irregular, which can put a strain on the heart muscle.

Valvular Heart Disease

Having valvular heart disease is a significant risk factor for AFib, to the point that often during valve surgery (open heart), the surgeon may empirically perform a maze procedure to reduce the chances of atrial fibrillation. As an aside, the maze procedure was first pioneered by Dr. James Cox in 1987, whereby the atria were compartmentalized through a series of incisions. If you imagine AFib as a group of disorganized cattle roaming freely, the idea behind the maze procedure was to fence off the cattle in different areas of the heart. Over time this has evolved from incisions to different types of ablation energy sources during surgery. Whether it is a leaky valve (regurgitation) or a narrowed valve (stenosis), both can result in increased pressure and size of the left and right atria, which can trigger AFib. If severe regurgitation or stenosis is present, it is paramount to treat these (medically or surgically when indicated) to reduce the chances of AFib alongside any specific rhythm control for AFib (drugs, ablation, etc.).

Athleticism as a Risk Factor

A growing group of high-endurance athletes are getting AFib in their forties and fifties. Several research groups have discovered that this may be due in part to an overactivated parasympathetic nervous system (PNS). The PNS—the counterbalance to the sympathetic or fight-or-flight response—is known to be a trigger for AFib. The PNS causes the heart rate to be low in endurance athletes.

A low heart rate can predispose you to premature atrial beats, which can trigger AFib. This is because it is easier for premature beats to arise when the heart rate is slower. As a result, many people with AFib experience episodes when they are relaxing rather than when they are active. When arrhythmias occur while you are at rest, you will be more aware of an abnormal heartbeat. This can create emotional and mental stress, leading to the brain's sympathetic nervous system sending more signals to the heart's electrical system. This becomes a vicious cycle. Because of these reasons, I usually recommend patients with premature beats to get up and move around—if they can. Movement increases your natural heartbeat (sinus node), which can overdrive and suppress the premature beats. The physical movement also releases endorphins, which can relieve stress and the resulting fight-or-flight response that can perpetuate arrhythmias.

Premature Atrial Contractions

It is now recognized that a high frequency of premature atrial contractions, known as PACs, can be a risk factor and trigger for AFib. This is best assessed on a twenty-four-hour Holter monitor. A PAC number of over 75 in a twenty-four-hour time period is considered frequent. In a 2013 study from the University of California San Francisco, frequent PACs increased the AFib risk up to 18 percent. One major hypothesis is that premature atrial beats can shorten the electrical recovery time of cells in the atria. This is called the atrial refractory period. By shortening this time, it is easier for several premature beats to occur in a row and trigger an episode of atrial fibrillation. Think of it as enough sparks to trigger a fire. Furthermore, premature atrial beats are often what trigger reentrant arrhythmias. Reentry is one of the three mechanisms of arrhythmias described earlier, similar to the idea of a merry-go-round that won't stop.

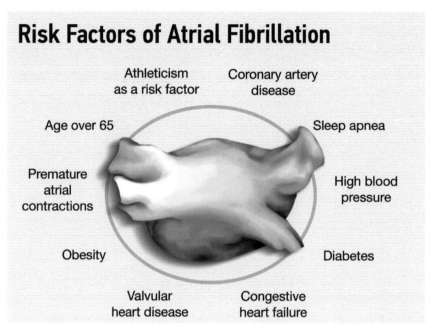

Risk Factors of Atrial Fibrillation

Athleticism as a risk factor

Coronary artery disease

Age over 65

Sleep apnea

Premature atrial contractions

High blood pressure

Obesity

Diabetes

Valvular heart disease

Congestive heart failure

Figure 8

We have traditionally told patients with premature beats that they are "benign." In a patient at risk for AFib, however, having a high frequency of premature beats may increase the likelihood of triggering an AFib event.

The first steps in lowering the count are to take a magnesium supplement; reduce or eliminate alcohol, caffeine, and any other stimulants; regular aerobic exercise; and stress management.

Atrial Fibrillation Triggers

ALCOHOL

While alcohol does not actually cause the AFib disease, it is a significant trigger for specific episodes. The reason is threefold: (1)

alcohol has a direct effect on the electrical system (holiday heart), (2) it causes dehydration (diuretic effect), and (3) it depletes the body of magnesium. People often ask if alcohol must be completely avoided. I always tell them that it should be avoided as much as possible. Why take the chance? Most of the time, people are attracted to the ritual of drinking a glass of wine at the end of the day or they are part of social circles that tend to drink together. If you *really* want that glass of wine, I recommend taking an additional magnesium supplement and drinking a lot of water.

CAFFEINE

The same basic principles regarding alcohol apply to caffeine. Caffeine is essentially a form of adrenaline, which can cause premature atrial beats that can trigger atrial fibrillation. Like alcohol, it has a diuretic/dehydration effect and also depletes the body of magnesium. If you really want to enjoy a morning coffee, decaf is usually okay. Although it has a small amount of caffeine, it is not usually enough to trigger arrhythmias.

Bottom line—listen to your body. If you start experiencing severe palpitations, identify the trigger and stop it.

ELECTROLYTE DEFICIENCY

The big electrolyte deficiencies are magnesium and potassium. Most of the body's stores of these electrolytes are located in tissue, not the bloodstream. For this reason, a serum (blood) level of magnesium and potassium do not truly reflect the body's state of deficiency. A normal level does not mean a person isn't deficient. For this reason, we typically recommend magnesium supplementation to all our patients—regardless of blood level—as long as they do not have advanced kidney disease.

As far as types go, some magnesiums are well absorbed by the body, and some are poorly absorbed. Good types include magnesium malate, citrate, glycinate, and taurate. Avoid magnesium oxide or gluconate. I often recommend Natural Vitality's Calm Gummies (two to four gummies per day), because chewing a gummy is often preferable to swallowing a "horse" pill (these supplements often come in the form of very large pills). You can find them online (at amazon.com or naturalvitality.com) or locally at health stores. On the West Coast, Sprouts carries them. Other good brands are Doctor's Best magnesium glycinate (200 mg once or twice a day) and Cardiovascular Research's magnesium taurate (125 mg twice a day). Taking magnesium at night helps with sleep and prevention of muscle cramps. If you get diarrhea or significant abdominal pain, try lowering the dose or changing to a different brand or type. For people intolerant of oral magnesium, magnesium oil spray is a great option. Ancient Minerals is a good brand for that.

One last point to note about magnesium is that there are some anecdotal reports of intravenous magnesium assisting in the conversion of atrial fibrillation to sinus rhythm. It is seen with other arrhythmias too, such as premature ventricular contractions and ventricular tachycardia. I treat a seventy-five-year-old man who has persistent atrial fibrillation. He has undergone two ablations and, for the most part, stays in sinus rhythm on relatively little medication. He has had some recurrences recently and he goes to a naturopath physician who runs an outpatient infusion center.

Here, patients can come in as walk-ins for IV magnesium therapy. There have been times where he was in AFib for up to seven days and required cardioversion to get him back into rhythm. There have been three instances when he went in after about three or four days of AFib, and within twenty-four to forty-eight hours of receiving magnesium he converted to sinus rhythm. Most recently, he went in for IV magnesium within twenty-four hours of the onset of AFib. He converted to sinus rhythm about twenty-four hours later. What is also interesting about him is that his serum magnesium levels are normal and he already takes a magnesium supplement. Since the diagnosis of AFib, he has gone to his naturopath about five times for magnesium infusions.

DEHYDRATION

Dehydration can be a trigger for AFib. The presumed mechanism is that adrenaline levels increase during states of dehydration because the body's goal is to maintain blood flow to vital organs. As mentioned, adrenaline has direct input into the heart's electrical system, so in this fashion, dehydration can trigger premature beats, which trigger AFib under the right circumstances. Often dehydration is coupled with electrolyte deficiency, as described above. It is not uncommon, for a person presenting to an emergency room with AFib, to have what is called an elevated blood urea nitrogen to creatinine ratio (BUN/Cr). An elevated ratio can indicate reduced blood flow to the kidneys, which can occur with dehydration. Other symptoms and signs of dehydration include dry mouth, reduced urine output, pale skin, and low blood pressure.

POOR SLEEP HYGIENE

Lack of sleep is typically not an independent trigger for AFib per se, but combined with dehydration, electrolyte deficiency, alcohol, caffeine, and stress, it can create the perfect-storm trigger for AFib. Sleep is such an important restorative aspect of our health. Getting proper sleep reduces cortisol and circulating levels of adrenaline. Both of these are involved in the stress response. Chronic sleep deprivation leads to increased stress hormone levels, including cortisol and adrenaline, which in turn can increase blood pressure and heart rate.

Regarding insomnia, there are several non-drug approaches to try first. Magnesium supplements that also help with arrhythmias can be taken. And taking a warm bath or shower at bedtime relaxes the body. You should avoid caffeine after 12 p.m. Sleep monitors have shown that caffeine affects sleep when consumed up to ten hours before sleep. Journaling is a mind-gentling activity. A mindfulness practice is another effective first-step approach to alleviating insomnia.

Also, try to exercise earlier in the day. Exercising right before bedtime can sometimes impair sleep, since adrenaline levels are high. Definitely avoid any screen time (phone, computer, TV) within an hour or so before bedtime. Reading a light book before bedtime can also help you turn off your mind. Regarding supplements, melatonin is generally safe and nonaddictive. There are supplements that also incorporate other components that can help with sleep, such as tryptophan, serotonin modifiers, and gamma-aminobutyric acid (GABA) modifiers.

Poor sleep is associated with a shorter lifespan, reduced

reproductive capability, reduced immunity, increased risk for cancer and cardiovascular disease, and accelerated cognitive decline. Regarding cardiovascular disease, consider that with the loss of an hour in the spring due to daylight savings time, there is a 40 percent increase in the number of heart attacks the following day.

For an informative TED talk on sleep by brain scientist Matt Walker, see:

https://www.ted.com/talks/matt_walker_sleep_is_your_superpower.

STRESS

People often ask me, "Can stress cause AFib?" First, it is important to make the distinction between a cause of AFib and a trigger for an AFib episode. Stress, through elevated adrenaline, can lead to premature beats, which can trigger AFib. However, usually emotional/mental stress alone is not enough to trigger AFib. Often it is in combination with other factors, such as dehydration or alcohol/caffeine.

The role of the autonomic nervous system is being increasingly recognized as a significant part of triggering and maintaining AFib. Stress triggers our fight-or-flight response and activates the sympathetic nervous system. Stress management techniques, such as breathing exercises or mindfulness practices, can help reduce the anxiety associated with palpitations and AFib. Can these techniques actually stop an episode? There is no data to suggest that.

However, I have seen countless people go to the ER with AFib lasting several hours, and as they are preparing for electrical cardioversion, they all of a sudden self-convert to normal sinus rhythm. Many have had an AFib at home but convert to sinus rhythm in the waiting room. My hypothesis is that when people arrive at a hospital, their stress is relieved because they know they will be taken care of and are in a safe place. It is well known that stress reduction reduces blood pressure and heart rate. So, I think that acutely reducing stress may have several beneficial effects when it comes to AFib.

In an era when we are constantly barraged with new sources of entertainment or news, and when the phone in our pocket or purse calls us to attention, we have ceded the spaces of quiet in our lives. It can be helpful to set aside a bit of truly quiet time each day, even if only a small period where our phone is turned off and we are listening only to our own quiet. Alan Watts, in his book *Still the Mind*, writes, "There is only now; there never was any time but now, and there never will be any time but now. It is all now. There is no hurry to gobble life down . . . so it's all right to just sit and be in the present."

EXERCISE

What?! How can exercise possibly be a trigger for AFib? Isn't it something that we doctors are always telling you to do? Well, first note that it does not happen often, but there are cases of what is called "adrenergic AFib," which is when exercise can trigger an AFib episode. Patients with adrenergic AFib often respond well to beta-blocker medication. However, the beta-blocker also blunts the heart-rate response to exercise, which can translate into feeling like you don't have as much endurance when exercising.

Conversely, vagally triggered AFib, the AFib that is often triggered by a low pulse rate, can sometimes convert to sinus rhythm when someone exercises. I would only advocate exercise, in the setting of AFib, after you are properly evaluated by an electrophysiologist, who suggests doing this. If your heart rate is already fast in AFib, and you exercise, it can increase to the point of dropping your blood pressure and this can cause you to faint. Nonetheless, there is a real entity of vagal AFib that terminates with exercise.

TIME OF DAY

It is not uncommon for people to report more AFib at night than during the day. There are several postulated mechanisms for this. The first is that the heart rate naturally slows at night due to the vagus nerve/parasympathetic nervous system. This is meant to be protective to the body and conserve energy because there is no reason why the body should work hard during restful states. When the heart rate slows, it is often easier for premature atrial beats to become triggered because there is a longer time interval between normal beats. This gives premature beat foci "more opportunity" to fire.

Conversely, AFib can be less frequent during the day, because your sinus node heart rate naturally suppresses premature beats. The second possible reason for the nocturnal predilection is stress. Often during the day, our minds are distracted and busy. At night, our thoughts can sometimes increase significantly when thinking about our worries, because there is nothing else to distract our minds. This can then trigger the sympathetic nervous system.

EATING

Believe it or not, eating or drinking can sometimes trigger AFib. Very hot or very cold liquids and large fatty meals are all notorious for triggering AFib in patients with a history of vagal triggers. There are two reasons for this. First, the esophagus and the heart are adjacent structures, so physical stimulation from one organ to another can occur. Second, the vagus nerve, the main component of the parasympathetic nervous system, has direct electrical input into both the gastrointestinal tract and the cardiovascular system. Because of this, electrical signals in one organ system can affect the other. I treat a forty-two-year-old triathlete patient named Johnny, who reported that he consistently went into AFib at the end of a race when he drank a cold Gatorade at the finish line.

Sean, a fifty-eight-year-old electrical engineer, recently reported having AFib episodes triggered by eating large, heavy meals in the evening. Usually, the episode would occur after he went to sleep. This meant there was typically a three-to-four-hour delay from the meal to the AFib episode. His AFib episodes would usually occur in the middle of the night, likely from a prominent vagal mechanism. While eliminating these types of triggers may not eliminate AFib, it certainly may reduce the frequency of episodes. As I have mentioned before and will mention again: *AFib begets AFib and sinus rhythm begets sinus rhythm.*

The Perfect Storm

People living with AFib often ask, "Why did I go into AFib then?" In my experience, I have often found that taking a careful history of the events leading up to an AFib episode can be quite revealing. There is always a chain of events involving some permutation of triggers that cause the perfect storm, so to speak.

Susan, a forty-five-year-old armed services veteran, describes it this way: "I have been very stressed out these last few months due to a family member being quite ill. I was out at dinner and had two glasses of wine. I ate a large portion of the main course and felt bloated after. Now that I think about it, I didn't have that much water to drink earlier in the day. I take hydrochlorothiazide for high blood pressure, which is a diuretic. I don't typically take a potassium or magnesium supplement." In this example, there is a mix of factors outside the patient's control and factors within the patient's control. Although everything cannot be controlled, eliminating some of the triggers will lessen the chances of a perfect storm and manage to stop a potential episode of AFib.

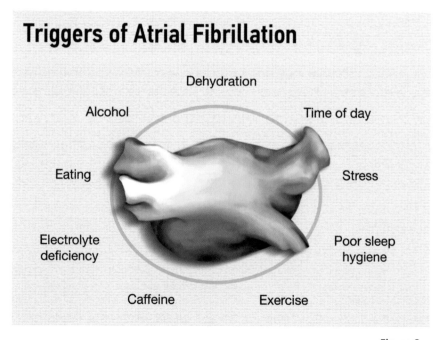

Triggers of Atrial Fibrillation

Dehydration

Alcohol

Time of day

Eating

Stress

Electrolyte deficiency

Poor sleep hygiene

Caffeine

Exercise

Figure 9

Self-Assessment:
AFib Risk Factors

A critical part of overcoming AFib is to identify what risk factors you have, assess their status, and work to optimize them. You want to create an achievable set of goals in managing these risk factors. Remember, by picking up this book, you have already overcome one of the greatest hurdles we can face with our health...starting the journey. Also, remember that optimizing these risk factors will have health benefits significantly beyond overcoming AFib: improved mood, sleep, well-being, and longevity. This is a process—not a race to the finish.

A practical matter: I recommend making several blank copies of the self-assessment sections, which you can use along your journey to overcome AFib. Your goals may change, your targets may change, or your priorities may change.

Place checkmarks, circle, and fill in the blanks as indicated:

Risk Factors

Yes No

___ ___ **Age over 65**

___ ___ **Obesity**

Current weight: _____ pounds, BMI: _____kg/m2.

Goal weight: _____ pounds, BMI: _____ kg/m2.

For the next 21 days, starting, __ /__ /__, I will exercise _____ min per day.

For the next 21 days, starting, __ /__ /__, I will eliminate (circle all that apply): pasta, bread, alcohol, fried foods, sweets, red meat.

___ ___ **High blood pressure**

Current average BP: ___ /___.

Goal average BP: ___ /___.

Salt intake: _____ grams per day.

For the next 21 days, starting __ /__ /__, I will reduce salt intake to _____ grams per day.

___ ___ **Sleep apnea**

I have the following (circle all that apply): snoring, sleepiness, witnessed apnea.

I have sleep apnea diagnosed by: ___ home apnea link, ___ formal sleep study.

Self-Assessment:
AFib Risk Factors (continued)

Risk Factors (continued)

Yes No

___ ___ **Sleep apnea** (continued)
My current treatment is:
___ CPAP, ___ dental appliance, ___ surgery.
I do not have a treatment plan for sleep apnea.
For the next 21 days, starting __ / __ / __, I will use
_____ for my sleep apnea.

___ ___ **Diabetes**
Current average blood sugar: _____.
Current hemoglobin A1c: _____.
Goal blood sugar: _____.
Goal hemoglobin A1c: _____.

___ ___ **Coronary artery disease**
Current total cholesterol _____.
Goal total cholesterol _____.
Last stress test __ / __ / __.

___ ___ **Congestive heart failure**
Current salt intake: _____ grams per day.
For the next 21 days, starting __ / __ / __, I will reduce salt
intake to _____ grams per day.

___ ___ **Valvular heart disease** (circle all that apply)
Valves affected: aortic, mitral, pulmonic, tricuspid.
Type of valve disease: stenosis, regurgitation, both.
Valve replacement: mechanical, bioprosthetic.
Last echo: __ / __ / __.

___ ___ **Athleticism**
My AFib is associated with this type of activity:
_____.
My AFib is associated with this heart rate: _____ bpm.

___ ___ **Premature atrial contractions**
Last Holter monitor: __ / __ / __.
PAC burden (%): _____.

Self-assessment: AFib Risk Factors

Self-Assessment:
AFib Risk Factors (continued)

After you have reviewed this list and entered in some data, I encourage you to share the list with a family member, friend, or health care provider. That makes it real. That creates an added level of accountability, which may be just what you need to stick to the plan and achieve your goals. Remember, this is not an all-inclusive list. You can do additional reading and research on all the risk factors for AFib to see what else you can optimize.

Notes

_____

_____

_____

_____

_____

_____

_____

_____

_____

_____

_____

_____

_____

_____

_____

_____

_____

_____

_____

Self-Assessment: AFib Triggers

Just as important as risk factors are the triggers for specific AFib episodes. In a similar fashion, you want to identify all the triggers you can think of, assess their status in your life (frequency of occurrence and predictability), and work to reduce the chances they will trigger AFib. Similar to risk factors, you want to do an inventory of your health and make a list of the triggers you have (and may not realize you have!). Second, you want to create an achievable set of goals in managing these triggers. This means reducing (eliminating if possible) alcohol and caffeine, staying well hydrated, taking electrolyte supplements, improving sleep hygiene and stress management techniques, charting any triggers related to activity level or time of day, and identifying the perfect-storm formula of factors that result in triggering a specific episode. Remember, by picking up this book, you have already overcome one of the greatest hurdles we can face with our health...starting the journey. Also, remember that optimizing these triggers will have health benefits significantly beyond overcoming AFib: improved mood, sleep, well-being, and longevity. This is a process—not a race to the finish.

A practical matter: I recommend making several blank copies of the self-assessment sections, which you can use along your journey to overcome AFib. Your goals may change, your targets may change, or your priorities may change.

Place checkmarks, circle, and fill in the blanks as indicated:

List of Triggers

Yes No

___ ___ **Alcohol**
I currently drink _____ ounces of beer/wine/hard liquor, _____ times, per (circle one) day/week/month.
For the next 21 days, starting __ / __ / __, I will (pick one):
☐ Eliminate it.
☐ Reduce it by _____ ounce(s), every _____ week.

___ ___ **Caffeine**
I currently drink _____ ounces of coffee/tea/soft drink, _____ times, per (circle one) day/week/month.
For the next 21 days, starting __ / __ / __, I will (pick one):
☐ Eliminate it.
☐ Reduce it by _____ ounce(s), every _____ week.

Self-Assessment: AFib Triggers (continued)

⚠️ **List of Triggers** (continued)

Yes No

___ ___ **Dehydration**
I currently drink _____ ounces of water, _____ times,
per (circle one) day/week/month.
For the next 21 days starting __ / __ / __, I will increase it
by _____ ounce(s), every _____ week.

___ ___ **Electrolyte deficiency**
For the next 21 days, starting __ / __ / __, I will take _____
milligram(s) of magnesium.

___ ___ **Poor sleep hygiene**
For the next 21 days, starting __ / __ / __, I will go to bed
by ___:___ p.m. and wake up by ___:___ a.m.

___ ___ **Stress**
For the next 21 days, starting __ / __ / __, I will do _____
(circle one) minute(s)/day(s) of mindfulness.

___ ___ **Exercise**
For the next 21 days, starting __ / __ / __, I will do _____
minute(s)/day(s) of the following: (circle all that apply)
walking/jogging/running/swimming/yoga/sports/
_____.

___ ___ **Time of day**
My AFib episodes often occur during this time of day:
(circle one) morning/afternoon/evening.

___ ___ **Eating**
My AFib episodes often occur when I eat/drink _____
_____.

Self-Assessment: AFib Triggers (continued)

List of Triggers (continued)

Yes No

____ ____ Eating (continued)
For the next 21 days, starting ___ / ___ / ___, I will avoid
eating/drinking _____.

____ ____ Perfect storm
Combination of _____, _____, _____.
For the next 21 days, starting ___ / ___ / ___, I will avoid
_____, _____, _____.

After you have reviewed this list and entered in some data, I encourage you to share with a family member, friend, or health care provider. That makes it real. That creates an added level of accountability, which may be just what you need to stick to the plan and achieve your goals. Remember, this is not an all-inclusive list. You can do additional reading and research on all the risk factors for AFib to see what else you can optimize.

Notes

_____
_____
_____
_____
_____
_____
_____
_____
_____
_____
_____
_____
_____
_____
_____
_____

CHAPTER 2

Confirmation

"Teach your tongue to say 'I do not know'
and you will progress."

—**Maimonides,** philosopher

"I personally am one of 5.8 million Americans who have
AFib not caused by a heart valve problem. And then when
I learned the facts, that this could possibly cause a stroke,
I thought, I better educate myself and go for help."

—**Howie Mandel,** TV host and comedian

Diagnosis of Atrial Fibrillation

The diagnosis of atrial fibrillation can be challenging. AFib can have a vast array of symptoms, or no symptoms at all. Early in the disease (paroxysmal AFib, or PAF), episodes and symptoms come and go. People tend to have symptoms of palpitations, which is a feeling that the heartbeat is irregular and fast. Since the episodes come and go, you may show up at your doctor's office in a normal rhythm with a normal EKG, so it is difficult to diagnose the problem (this occurs quite commonly). Furthermore, even people with PAF can have asymptomatic episodes (called "silent AFib"), especially at night while sleeping. This phenomenon was first demonstrated in research studies about pacemaker patients with PAF. Most modern pacemakers have sophisticated algorithms to record very short episodes of AFib, which often are asymptomatic. Showing up in a normal rhythm, or being in a normal rhythm during the entire time you wear a heart rhythm monitor, is akin to taking your car to the mechanic but then being told it doesn't "act up" at the shop.

It is important to mention that patients with PAF, and other arrhythmias such as supraventricular tachycardia, can be diagnosed as having panic attacks if they were in AFib at home but by the time they arrived at the emergency room they had already converted to sinus rhythm. When you are in AFib, it is normal to feel anxious and unsettled because the heart rate is often going very fast. One of the key differences between an arrhythmia causing those symptoms versus a true anxiety attack is that often with AFib a person may not be feeling anxious or stressed when the event occurs. This is in contrast to a true anxiety attack, where often a specific situation or set of circumstances provokes the response.

Persistent atrial fibrillation, which is continuous atrial fibrillation occurring for more than seven days consecutively, can be much more subtle in the way of symptoms. The most common symptoms include fatigue, malaise, and an overall sense of not feeling well. In fact, people often don't realize they are having symptoms until normal sinus rhythm is restored. Symptoms of racing heartbeat, chest discomfort, or shortness of breath may be absent. If the main symptom is a reduction in exercise tolerance, a person may adjust their physical activity. Think of it like having arthritis in your knee. Rather than focus on the pain, you may just avoid activities that stress it. We call this phenomenon "accommodation." Then, your joint is repaired or replaced, and you now notice you are able to walk farther, climb stairs easily, and don't live with a background nagging discomfort you didn't realize was there. It is for this reason that electrophysiologists will often recommend a cardioversion procedure to restore the rhythm to see if a person feels any better. Even if normal sinus rhythm lasts one or two days, if a person feels better during that time, that is very helpful to know when it comes to devising a treatment strategy. This knowledge would typically mean that a rhythm-control strategy should be undertaken, in the form of a drug or an ablation.

In some cases, with AFib, a patient does not feel anything, but their spouse or partner may notice the skin is pale or that they fall asleep easily during the day. While daytime sleepiness can be a sign of sleep apnea, sometimes it is specifically a symptom of persistent AFib.

One of the most common scenarios for the diagnosis of persistent AFib is the pre-op physical or routine office visit. A patient, for example, planning to have gallbladder surgery, visits the doctor prior to the procedure and has an EKG during that visit. The

EKG shows AFib. The patient is then asked, "Have you had any palpitations or irregular heartbeat?" The answer is almost always no, because palpitations and irregular heartbeat are not what most people experience. The most common symptom of persistent AFib is actually fatigue. If a person is not physically active or is older, they may ascribe any fatigue to those factors, not necessarily AFib. It is often helpful to ask whether in the past six months to a year if there was a change in energy level or exercise tolerance. Furthermore, a person's spouse or partner can sometimes pick up on subtle cues such as a change in a person's facial complexion (they look paler due to reduced blood flow). When AFib is diagnosed, it is important to review all prior EKGs to see when the last documented normal sinus rhythm was present.

One of the most helpful measures of the duration of AFib is the size and volume of the left atrial chamber of the heart on a routine 2-D echocardiogram, or ultrasound of the heart. The longer and more frequent AFib a person has, the larger the chamber grows. Besides giving a sense of chronology, the size of the atrium has prognostic value in the long-term maintenance of sinus rhythm. For example, an atrium greater than 5.5 centimeters is associated with a low rate of sinus rhythm long term.

Cardiac MRI is another modality that can be helpful to determine chronicity of the arrhythmia. Magnetic resonance imaging is very good at detecting scar tissue in the heart. It was first used for assessment of the ventricles in patients who had had a prior heart attack (which creates scarring). Now there are software applications that allow imaging and processing of atrial tissue to determine the amount of scar present. Usually the more scarring there is, the larger the atrium. Since that is not always true, however, having cardiac MRI can be very helpful as another tool in the toolbox of diagnostic testing.

You Don't Know if You Don't Try

I recently encountered an incredible example of the varying array of symptoms with atrial fibrillation. At my office I saw Joe, a seventy-two-year-old gentleman with persistent atrial fibrillation. Joe spent most of his life serving his country as a United States Marine. He was a family man and would do anything for his friends. If anyone asked what kind of person Joe was, they would say he was vibrant and full of energy.

However, that is not who Joe was over the past year. He couldn't figure out why he felt zapped of energy even when he wasn't active. Joe also felt depressed—not enjoying all the good things he had in his life. He had a difficult time processing information and wondered if it was the early stage of dementia. Joe did not go to the doctor often, but at the urging of his wife of thirty-two years, he went. His physician detected an irregular pulse and the EKG showed atrial fibrillation. Joe was then referred to me for evaluation. Based on the time line of Joe's fatigue and depressive symptoms, I wondered whether AFib was the source of it all.

We did a cardiac workup and talked about treatment options. Joe wanted to try a noninvasive approach first, so we did a cardioversion. He converted to normal rhythm and felt like a different person. All the fatigue and depression resolved. The AFib recurred a week after the procedure, which is quite common with persistent AFib, especially if a patient is not on an antiarrhythmic drug or has had a prior ablation. With the recurrence of AFib, the fatigue, depression, and all the terrible symptoms accompanying it returned. In fact, interestingly enough, it was Joe's wife, Wanda, who first detected AFib was back. She noticed a fairly immediate change in Joe's color and demeanor.

I sat down with Joe and Wanda and first reassured them that they had several options available to them. I cannot emphasize this point enough. People need hope—realistic hope, but hope. When someone is told nothing can be done for their AFib, it is important to carefully examine all the data from the workup and try to establish if the AFib had caused any symptoms. In our discussion, antiarrhythmic drugs and ablation were presented. Joe did not want to take any more medication, and after reading the side effects and toxicities of the different antiarrhythmic drugs, he felt ablation was his best option. I also recommended ablation to Joe. He underwent a cryoballoon pulmonary vein isolation procedure in combination with a contact force-sensing radiofrequency ablation of right atrial cavo-tricuspid isthmus flutter and left atrial posterior wall isolation (these procedures are explained in more detail in Chapter 3). Joe converted to sinus rhythm at the end of the ablation procedure. The most impressive change is that he has much greater mental clarity. He also feels like the low-level depression he experienced for years has finally lifted. I told him it makes sense because his heart is now more efficient in pumping blood throughout the body, including the brain.

The Diagnostic Dilemma

The above discussion focused on persistent AFib symptoms. Paroxysmal AFib can be similar in some regards and different in others. As the name suggests, paroxysmal means that a patient's AFib starts and stops on its own. This can be associated with the abrupt onset of a racing or irregular pulse, or other symptoms that reflect poor blood flow through the body, such as lightheadedness, shortness of breath, chest discomfort, or general malaise. The difference with paroxysmal AFib is that there are typically discrete events or episodes of these symptoms and then other times a person feels completely fine. This is where heart-rhythm monitoring is critical to establish whether AFib is occurring and whether it correlates with any specific symptoms.

In many cases of paroxysmal AFib there is an associated feeling of anxiety or feeling unsettled. This is often due to the high adrenaline levels circulating in the body during an arrhythmia episode. I've seen many cases where people were misdiagnosed as having panic attacks because by the time they arrived at the emergency room for evaluation, the AFib episode had already terminated. The key here is that these "panic attacks" usually do not occur in response to a stressor. They often occur at rest when it is easier for premature atrial beats to trigger AFib, because the heart rate is slower at rest. This diagnosis of AFib as "panic attacks" often occurs in younger patients with the arrhythmia, who have no structural heart disease. Doctors may not suspect AFib because the patient has a normal heart.

Diagnosing problems with the heart's electrical system can be challenging because the malfunctioning circuits often "come and go." This is in contrast to the heart's coronary arteries, where a high-grade blockage is present continuously, so a stress test or angiogram often reveals the problem. Patients who ultimately get diagnosed with AFib often tell me, "This has never come up before when I go to my doctor's appointments." Again, because paroxysmal AFib comes and goes, on any given day at an office appointment the EKG may be normal. Keep in mind, the EKG is only a split second in time.

The key to making a heart-rhythm diagnosis is continuous rhythm monitoring with the ability to record symptoms in association with rhythm. That way we can establish whether a person's palpitations are due to a rhythm-based cause like premature beats, or whether they are due to other causes such as stress. Beyond symptom diagnosis, given the high incidence of silent AFib as a cause of stroke of unknown origin (cryptogenic stroke), it has become even more important to be able to detect asymptomatic AFib episodes with monitoring technology. Traditionally, there are five types of monitors: *Holter monitors* (continuous, up to forty-eight hours), *event recorders* (only symptom-activated, may miss asymptomatic AFib), *telemetry monitors* (continuous recording, real-time transmissions, require good cell signal), *patch monitors* (up to two weeks, no wires, waterproof, chip recording that does not transmit daily), and *implantable monitors* (continuous recording for up to three years). In the last few years we have seen significant improvements in wearable technology to monitor the heart's rhythm and help diagnose AFib. These include smartphone-based sensors and smartwatch-based sensors.

Let's discuss these different rhythm-monitoring methods in more detail.

Catching the Heart Rhythm

Holter Monitor

Often, when patients are referred to us electrophysiologists, they have already had some type of diagnostic testing of the electrical system. Usually, an EKG has already been done, and frequently a

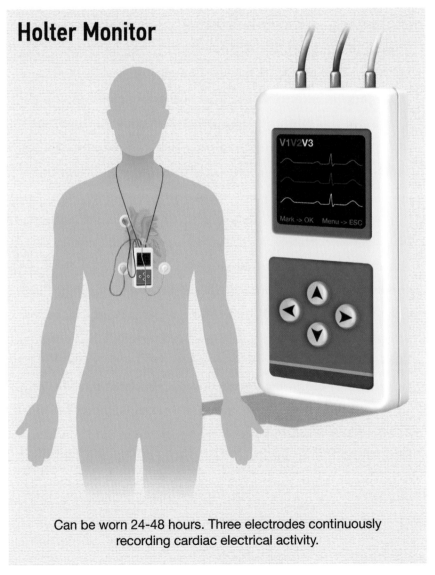

Holter Monitor

Can be worn 24-48 hours. Three electrodes continuously recording cardiac electrical activity.

Figure 10

Holter monitor has been worn by the patient. A Holter monitor consists of three electrodes and wires, which connect them to the recording device. Holter monitors typically are the largest of the monitoring devices, so they can be relatively bulky under clothing. A big advantage of Holter monitors is the continuous rhythm recording they offer. This has only a few applications, however.

Holter monitors have relatively low utility when it comes to diagnosing any cardiac arrhythmia, let alone AFib. This is because, as mentioned above, cardiac arrhythmias are often intermittent. If you think of statistics, monitoring for just twenty-four or forty-eight hours is unlikely to reveal the diagnosis. However, there is some value for Holter monitoring. For example, if a person is having daily palpitation symptoms, then one can use a continuous recording on a Holter to correlate a patient's symptoms with the heart's rhythm. But AFib rarely occurs daily.

Another use for a Holter monitor is to assess the adequacy of heart-rate control in a patient with permanent AFib. A heart rate of 60 to 80 beats per minute at rest and 110 to 120 beats per minute with exercise is considered reasonable. A resting heart rate that is fast, such as 130 to 140 beats per minute, can weaken the heart muscle over time. This is called a tachycardia mediated cardiomyopathy.

One more use of Holter monitoring, unrelated to AFib, is to assess the number of premature ventricular contractions (PVCs) in a twenty-four-hour time period, known as PVC burden. Here, a high burden of over 20 percent can be associated with the development of a different kind of weakening of the heart muscle called a PVC cardiomyopathy.

Event Recorder

In the time line of technology, Holter came first. Then came event recorders. These devices, like Holter, typically have three electrodes placed on the chest that are removable, for instance when someone showers. The electrodes are connected to wires, which are connected to the device. The device is typically smaller than a Holter. These devices can be worn longer than a Holter (the Holter limit is forty-eight hours). Typically, insurance will cover up to four weeks of monitoring. The goal with these monitors is to correlate symptom with rhythm. They are useful in making a rhythm diagnosis or ruling out one. As far as AFib is concerned, electrophysiologists tend not to order this type of monitor, because we want to see all episodes of AFib, ones that are symptomatic and ones that are asymptomatic (silent AFib). These monitors often have some limited retrograde and antegrade monitoring capability. What that means is that if someone has an abnormal heart rhythm associated with the symptom, there is sometimes a brief recording before and after the symptom-activated button is pushed.

The goal here is to "catch" the beginning (termed onset) and ending (termed offset or termination) of the arrhythmia. These monitors have limited ability to do this, however. Ultimately, event recorders have largely been replaced by patch monitors or telemetry monitors because both of those allow for symptom-activated triggers. As well, they also continuously record and apply certain algorithms to detect arrhythmias including silent AFib. Some insurances will not cover patch or telemetry monitors, making either a Holter or event recorder the only options. But the vast majority of insurances including Medicare cover patch and telemetry monitors.

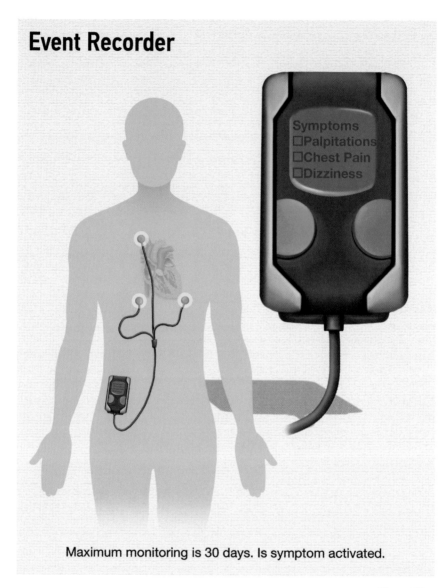

Event Recorder

Symptoms
☐Palpitations
☐Chest Pain
☐Dizziness

Maximum monitoring is 30 days. Is symptom activated.

Figure 11

Telemetry Monitor

Telemetry monitors are one step forward from event recorders. Usually, the maximum monitoring duration is four weeks. This can be shorter or extended, depending on the circumstances and insurance coverage. These monitors typically have three electrodes

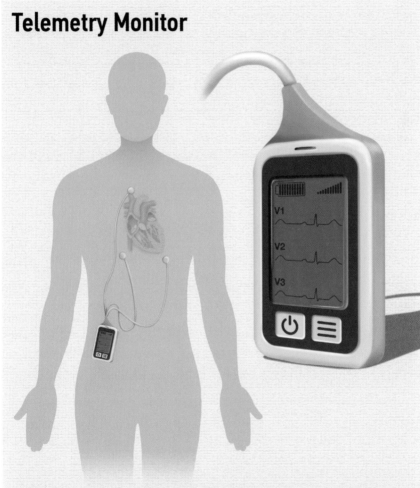

Maximum monitoring is 30 days. Provides real-time upload of rhythm data to central monitoring service, which will notify care provider based on alert criteria. Typically uses a cell signal to transmit information. Can detect silent and symptomatic arrhythmias.

Figure 12

connected to the device via three wires. The device is usually smaller than a Holter, and the electrodes and device are removable. A cell phone–type unit is worn, which transmits rhythm information in real time via cell phone networks to a central monitoring company. This occurs whether a patient has symptoms or not. What that means is there is an algorithm designed to automatically detect certain arrhythmias that meet certain criteria. These criteria, which are adjustable by the physician, include pauses over three seconds, heart rate over a certain threshold (usually more than 150 bpm), and irregularity in heart rhythm (the hallmark of AFib—so they can detect silent AFib). These monitors are typically chosen when a health care provider wants to know in real time whether someone is having a symptomatic or silent arrhythmia.

These monitors do not 100-percent diagnose a rhythm problem; they simply identify the possibility of one. If someone is exercising and the heart rate exceeds the detection threshold, it may be flagged as an arrhythmia. Similarly, if someone is in normal sinus rhythm but having a lot of extra beats, such as PACs or PVCs, it may get flagged as possible AFib.

Lastly, if there is a loss of electrode contact that creates noise on the tracing, it could be flagged as a pause or an arrhythmia. This is why there is a central monitoring company where staff members screen the transmissions to determine whether true arrhythmia is present or if it is just a false positive. Physicians can choose how to be notified in real time: email, call, or fax. Because monitoring typically is 24/7, if someone has an arrhythmia in the middle of the night, a health care provider can be notified immediately. A limitation of this type of monitor is cell phone signal availability. If there are limited networks in a patient's area, there may be problems with the signal transmission, which can be detrimental to the patient and the health care provider.

Patch Monitor

The advent of patch monitors was a major step forward in outpatient rhythm monitoring. Here, a device that looks like a large Band-Aid is applied to the skin over the heart region on the chest. It has two electrodes, which do a good job recording high-quality signals from the heart. Two big advantages exist with these monitors: They are typically water-resistant, which means they do not have to be removed to shower, and there are no wires involved, so they are less detectable and more comfortable. Many patients prefer to wear these monitors.

The big limitation, however, is that these monitors do not actively transmit data on a day-to-day basis. They record the rhythm on a chip within the device. At the end of the monitoring period, the device is removed and mailed to the monitoring company in a provided envelope. Usually, the maximum duration of monitoring is two weeks. The data is analyzed by people trained in arrhythmia diagnosis and a detailed report is sent to the physician, as a hard copy and online.

The turnaround for report generation is usually seven days. This means that a physician cannot diagnose your symptoms in real time, because they will not get the data until the monitor is turned in. This is especially relevant in the setting of AFib. If one is not on a blood thinner to protect against stroke, and the device shows AFib, the data will not be immediately available. So, we do not recommend this type of monitor when real-time decisions are being made about starting a blood thinner, in a patient deemed at high risk for stroke with AFib.

Patch Monitor

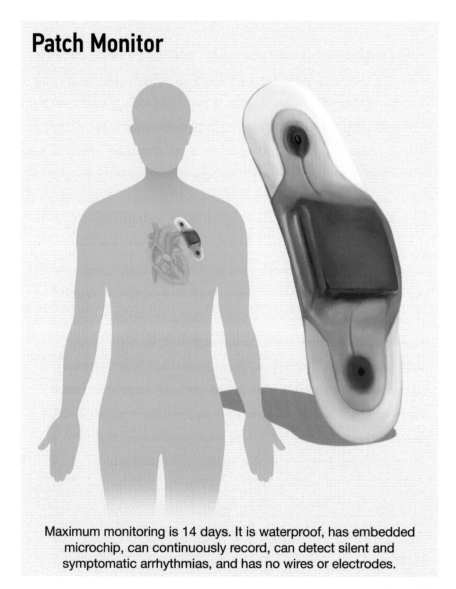

Maximum monitoring is 14 days. It is waterproof, has embedded microchip, can continuously record, can detect silent and symptomatic arrhythmias, and has no wires or electrodes.

Figure 13

Implantable Monitor

The implantable rhythm monitor is one of the greatest advancements in diagnosing both symptomatic and silent cardiac arrhythmias. These monitors have been around for a few decades. The original types were fairly large and required a surgical procedure to implant. Over the last several years, the monitors have been downsized significantly so they are essentially "injected" under the skin.

They are close to the size of a matchstick. Only a local anesthetic is required and sedation is usually not needed. Just recently, the FDA has approved implanting these in an office-type setting as long as certain infection-control criteria are met. At the vast majority of institutions, they are typically implanted in a hospital setting either in the same-day care unit or the catheterization lab. They can also be implanted at the time of an ablation procedure. Regardless of location, the implant takes only a few minutes. There are several advantages to this monitoring technology. The battery life is usually around three years, which means this is a great option for people who have infrequent symptoms. A four-week monitor will unlikely catch an arrhythmia if symptoms only occur a few times a year. The algorithms for autodetection of pauses, AFib, and other arrhythmias are fairly sophisticated.

Usually, these devices come with a base unit, which is plugged in next to a bed. They are usually programmed to do an automatic upload in the middle of the night or early morning. Here, an office or device clinic will get data about any symptomatic or asymptomatic arrhythmia events within twenty-four hours during the business week or on Mondays after the weekend. The base station can be taken when someone goes out of town for an extended period of time. However, the device will continue to monitor even without the base station and will transmit once it is within a certain distance of the monitor. For example, if you traveled to Italy for two weeks and had three episodes of AFib, once you return and are near the monitor, it will upload that information and send it to the doctor's office. Data is uploaded via cell phone towers, so the device can transmit wherever there is a cell phone signal.

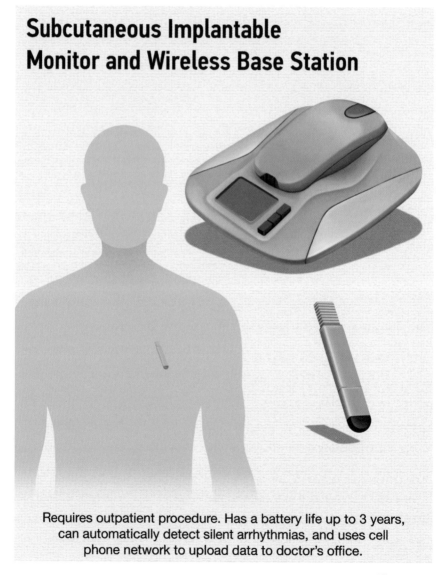

Subcutaneous Implantable Monitor and Wireless Base Station

Requires outpatient procedure. Has a battery life up to 3 years, can automatically detect silent arrhythmias, and uses cell phone network to upload data to doctor's office.

Figure 14

If there are several arrhythmia events during those two weeks, only the most recent will be recorded, depending on the memory storage of the device. This device is very attractive for both patient and physician, because patients don't have to think about their heart rhythm and physicians can have greater confidence in catching cardiac arrhythmias. These monitors are also useful for diagnosing unexplained fainting, called syncope. Again, because of the auto-detection algorithms, if someone faints and has a four-second pause that led to it, the device will identify the pause without the patient needing to record anything. This is especially useful when someone does not have warning symptoms before fainting.

Smartphone-Enabled and Smartwatch Monitors

Currently, there is a rapidly growing market of smartphone-enabled and smartwatch monitors that record the heart's rhythm. These are beyond conventional devices, which only record the heart rate. The first device that allowed for rhythm monitoring was the Kardia device by AliveCor. It utilizes a small finger pad, which has a Bluetooth interface with the smartphone. When patients want to do a recording, they do so using the finger pad and phone. One limitation is that you have to carry the finger pad with you, if your symptoms are unpredictable or episodic.

A recent development in smartwatch technology has allowed the ability to record a single-lead EKG such that it is much more portable than a smartphone/finger-pad system. This is the Apple Watch Series 4. To give an example, I was recently stopped in the hospital hallway by one of our doctors who performs anesthesia for our ablation procedures. He is a big fan of Apple products and

Smartphone-Enabled Monitor

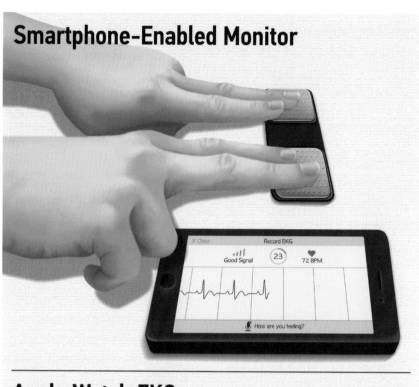

Apple Watch EKG

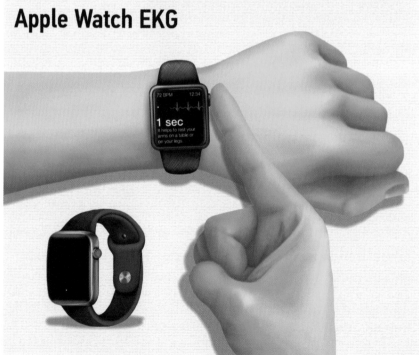

Figure 15

recently got the new Apple Watch Series 4 with the EKG feature. He was experiencing palpitations while driving his car and pulled over to do a recording. He showed me the EKG tracing and I was astounded by how clean and clear the signal was. I could see clearly organized atrial beats (sinus rhythm) and every other heartbeat was premature (premature atrial contraction). On a regular blood-pressure machine or Fitbit-type watch, only a pulse or irregular heartbeat sign would show. This tracing from the Apple Watch was as good as a rhythm monitor. And he could display it clearly on his iPad for me to review.

As you can see from the above descriptions of rhythm monitor technology, there are multiple ways to diagnose cardiac arrhythmias, including AFib. The choice is dependent on the frequency of symptoms, whether silent episodes need to be recorded, and ease of patient use.

Remember, once a diagnosis of atrial fibrillation is confirmed, you need to become informed. That means finding out what the disease is, what could be contributing to you developing it (health conditions, lifestyle factors), and what your options for treatment are. Remember, no two people with AFib are alike, just as no two people generally are alike.

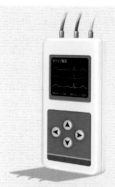

Holter Monitor

· 24-48 hours of continuous recording
· 3-5 electrodes and wires
· Useful to assess heart rate control for patients with persistent and permanent AFib
· Other applications: assess premature ventricular contraction burden, correlate daily symptoms with rhythm

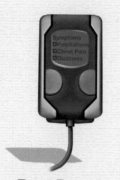

Event Recorder

· Up to 30 days of recording
· Smaller than Holter
· 3 removable electrodes and wires
· Symptom activated (not for silent arrhythmias)
· Limited antegrade and retrograde monitoring

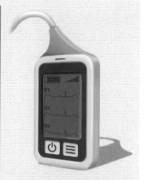

Telemetry Monitor

· Up to 30 days of recording
· Data transmitted to central monitoring service
· Requires adequate cell signal for data transmission
· Smaller than Holter
· 3 removable electrodes and wires
· Continuous monitoring (good for silent arrhythmia detection)

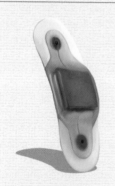

Patch Monitor

· Up to 14 days of continuous monitoring
· Waterproof "Band-Aid" with embedded chip that records rhythm
· Does not transmit data in real time - chip is processed at end of monitoring period

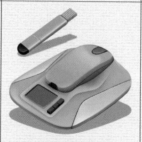

Subcutaneous Implantable Monitor and Wireless Base Station

· Up to 3 years of rhythm monitoring
· "Injected" under skin over left chest region
· Automatically uploads rhythm data to base unit
· Base unit transmits information via cell networks to doctor's office
· Manual data transmission optional

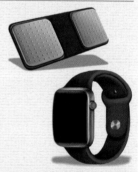

Smartphone-Enabled and Watch Monitors

· Fingers placed on bluetooth enabled pad with electrodes (smartphone-enabled)
· Watch automatically detects changes in rate and rhythm
· Watch can do manual EKG recording with finger sensor

Figure 16

Questions to Ask Your AFib Specialist - Part 1 of 2

? What is AFib?

How serious is my AFib and will it get better?

_____

_____

How long have I had AFib?

_____

_____

Why do I not feel symptoms of my AFib?

_____

_____

Is there an intensity factor to AFib or is it just on or off?

_____

_____

In what ways does AFib increase my health risks?

_____

_____

Do I have other health concerns that may increase my risk?

_____

_____

Am I at risk for a stroke? _____

✓ Testing

Do you recommend additional testing?

_____

_____

Do I have an electrolyte imbalance?

_____

_____

Lifestyle Changes

Do I need to make lifestyle changes? _____

Should I change any of the following to reduce my risks:

Eating habits?_____

_____

Physical activity? _____

_____

Smoking habits? _____

_____

Weight? _____

Questions to Ask Your AFib Specialist - Part 2 of 2

+ Medications & Treatments

What are medication options?

_____

_____

_____

What should I expect from it?

_____

_____

_____

What are other treatments?

_____

_____

_____

Should I be taking magnesium?

_____

_____

_____

Which blood thinner is the best?

_____

_____

_____

Will I need an ablation procedure in the future?

_____

_____

_____

When should these other options be considered?

_____

_____

_____

With my treatment plan, what should I expect to see?

_____

_____

_____

What are my treatment goals?

_____

Should I be taking a medication for AFib?

_____

_____

What will happen if I don't take the medication?

_____

_____

What are my other possible options?

_____

_____

Will I need blood thinners in the future?

_____

_____

What rhythm drug is the best and are they safe?

_____

_____

What are the risks and success rates of ablation?

_____

_____

When will we know that I am making progress with my treatment plan?

_____

_____

CHAPTER 3

Control

"The most difficult thing is the decision to act,
the rest is merely tenacity."
—**Amelia Earhart,** American aviation pioneer

"If anyone ever gets diagnosed with atrial fibrillation, just keep
plugging with it. Don't let it change what your goals are."
—**Karsten Madsen,** triathlete

Before we go into a discussion of the different treatment options for atrial fibrillation, let's again review the definition of "overcome" given in the Preface. It means "to succeed in dealing with a problem or difficulty." It does not necessarily mean cure. This chapter is about arming yourself with the knowledge to manage AFib so your life is not controlled by the condition, but rather you control your response to the challenge. As we mention throughout the book, "success" can mean something different to each person who has AFib.

For the person with early-onset paroxysmal AFib, this could mean the elimination of the arrhythmia through risk-factor modification, trigger modification, and/or catheter ablation. For the person with persistent AFib for less than one year, this could mean a reduction in symptomatic episodes so that quality of life improves. For a person with persistent AFib over one year (long-standing persistent AFib), this could mean the maintenance of normal sinus rhythm or a reduction of symptomatic episodes through a multitiered approach of drug therapy, ablative therapy, and device therapy. For someone with permanent AFib, in which sinus rhythm cannot be restored or where the risk of treatment is greater than the risk of disease, success could mean prevention of stroke via blood-thinner therapy or left atrial appendage occlusion therapy and control of the heart rate to prevent congestive heart failure and symptoms, which can impact quality of life. One of the most important things to keep in mind is that, because AFib is different person-to-person, one needs to be extremely careful about comparing results with others, in regard to treatment interventions.

The longer someone has AFib, and the more remodeling of the atria occurs (chamber enlargement, scarring), the greater the likelihood of recurrence. That being said, using a multitiered approach has helped many people with AFib. As EPs, one of our biggest challenges is making sure people have realistic expectations of what can be done to treat AFib and the success rates of the treatment interventions. I always tell my patients that maintaining sinus rhythm is about muscle memory.

Every day of sinus rhythm, the heart is remembering sinus rhythm.

In some regards, it doesn't matter how we get there: risk factor modification, trigger modification, risk factor plus trigger modification, ablation, ablation plus drug, ablation plus device, ablation plus drug plus device. If any of these alone or in combination result in a reduction of AFib, one could argue that is a success.

Remember, AFib is like electrical cancer. The more it spreads, the lower the chances of long-term maintenance of sinus rhythm. I often hear people say something like, "AFib ablation doesn't work. My friend had three and still has AFib." Well, if that friend has risk factors for AFib that are not being optimized—obesity, high blood pressure, alcohol intake—the AFib will continue regardless of ablation, drug, or device. Also, if that friend has severe left atrial enlargement because the disease had already progressed by the time the first ablation was done, there is going to be a higher recurrence rate. Lastly, if that friend had an ablation done five years ago, the technology at that time was inferior to the technology we have now. In some cases, this is about reframing your thinking about what it means to be successful in the treatment of your AFib.

Therapeutic Options for Atrial Fibrillation

I can't begin to tell you how often someone says, "My doctor said there's really nothing else to do except live in AFib." In fact, I just met with a patient in sinus rhythm after being in persistent AFib for three years. Jack is a sixty-five-year-old retired businessman who was absolutely miserable from AFib. (More about Jack later, in Case Studies.) We are using a combination of drug, ablation, and a pacemaker to treat his AFib.

He has maintained sinus rhythm through a combination of therapies: drug, ablation, and pacemaker. The point is, he is in sinus rhythm and that's what matters. When he was in AFib, his quality of life was like a home that was falling apart. And now, he has a new lease. As he was leaving the office recently, in sinus rhythm, he turned to me and said, "Three years ago I was told nothing could be done. Thankfully, I kept looking for someone who specialized in this."

The treatment of the disease is retraining the heart muscle to be in sinus rhythm, not AFib. While some patients may not be able to go back to life with sinus rhythm, that number has been shrinking due to two things: an increase in detection of AFib early on in the disease, and improvements in the treatment of AFib, in particular, catheter ablation. I am not saying everyone can be converted to sinus rhythm. What I am saying is that early detection and early intervention are critical with this disease, and mass education of health care professionals is desperately needed. Because AFib is not what it used to be when we learned about it in medical school, I will say it again: *mass education of health care professionals is needed*, because the treatment of AFib has improved tremendously, even within the last few years.

The Debate of Rhythm versus Rate Control

There are three principal strategies to manage atrial fibrillation: stroke prevention, rate control, and rhythm control. Stroke prevention will be covered later in this chapter. Regarding rate and rhythm control, there has been a debate in the field of electrophysiology as to whether a person's outcome is any different between a rate-control strategy and a rhythm-control strategy. Outcome is measured by all-cause mortality, cardiovascular mortality, hospitalizations, heart failure, stroke, recurrent AFib, and quality-of-life impact.

In 2002, a landmark clinical trial, called AFFIRM, randomized patients with AFib to rate-control versus rhythm-control strategies. No significant difference in mortality was observed. However, this trial included a very small number of patients who had ablation. Most of the rhythm-control patients were managed on antiarrhythmic drugs, which are known to have many toxicities, thereby negating the benefit of these drugs. Furthermore, many of the rhythm-control patients were taken off anticoagulation, putting them at higher risk of stroke.

Being in atrial fibrillation causes two negative physiologic effects on heart function: the loss of atrial "kick," which diminishes the amount of blood filling the ventricles and being pumped to the rest of the body, and a rapid irregular pulse, which limits the amount of filling in the ventricles that impacts the pump performance of the heart. It is for these two reasons that rhythm control is ideal. With rate control, the main goal is slowing the pulse. In some cases, an AV node ablation and pacemaker are used when medications are ineffective or not tolerated in controlling the heart rate. AV node ablation helps maintain a normal heart rate and regularizes the rhythm. Medications to control rate do not regularize the rhythm. Subsequent studies over the years with better ablation technologies have shown superiority of rhythm over rate control in several patient populations.

Let us now look at these two strategies in more detail.

Rhythm Control

Rhythm-control treatments of AFib beyond trigger and risk-factor modification include antiarrhythmic drugs, cardioversion, devices, and ablation.

ANTIARRHYTHMIC DRUGS

Medication for rhythm control includes what are called antiarrhythmic drugs. Several of these drugs have been around for decades. The challenge with drug therapy is the high incidence of side effects and toxicities. One of the biggest hurdles in drug development is trying to produce a therapy that is specific for atrial electrical tissue. Most of the existing drugs provide a "blanket" effect on the entire electrical system. This means that several drugs can cause arrhythmias (proarrhythmic) in addition to treating arrhythmias.

The challenge in atria-specific drugs partly lies in the nature of the electrical system. Because there are so many ion channels and factors involved in the electrical system, it is difficult to determine which channels need modification in a disease so heterogeneous as AFib. While there have been major milestones in other branches

AFib Antiarrhythmic Drugs

Class	Drug	Dose	Side effects	Serious reactions	Avoid use in	Can be used with
Sodium Channel Blockers — 1A	Disopyramide (Norpace)	Immediate release: 150mg every 6-8 hrs Controlled release: 150-300mg every 12 hrs	· Dry mouth · Dry eyes · Difficulty urinating	· CHF · Ventricular arrhythmias	· CHF · Glaucoma · Urinary retention	· Vagal atrial fibrillation · Hypertrophic cardiomyopathy
1C	Flecainide (Tambocor)*	50-150mg 2x daily	· Headache · Dizziness	· Ventricular arrhythmias · AV block	· Structural heart disease · Patients on digoxin	· Patients without structural heart disease
	Propafenone (Rhythmol)	Immediate release: 150-300mg every 8 hrs Extended release: 225-425mg every 12 hrs	· Dizziness · Taste changes · Nausea · Slow heart rate · Fatigue	· AV block · Ventricular arrhythmias · CHF	· Structural heart disease	· Patients without structural heart disease
III (potassium channel blockers)	Amiodarone (Pacerone)	100-200mg daily	· Fatigue, nausea · Tremor · Photosensitivity · Dizziness · Slow heart rate · Hypo-/hyper-thyroidism · Corneal deposits	· Liver toxicity · Lung toxicity · AV block	· Patients <50y.o. · Lung disease · Thyroid disorders · Liver disorders · Slow heart rate	· CHF · CM · CAD · VHD
	Dronedarone (Multaq)	400mg 2x daily	· GI upset (take with food) · Rash	· CHF · AV block	· CHF · Slow heart rate	· CAD · VHD · Lung disease
	Sotalol (Betapace)	80-160mg 2x daily	· Fatigue · Dizziness · Sleep disturbance · Depression · Erectile dysfunction · Hair loss · Wheezing	· VA-QT · CHF · AV block	· CHF · Prolonged QT interval · Slow heart rate · Asthma/lung disease · Depression · LVH	· VHD · CAD
	Dofetilide (Tikosyn)	125 - 500 mcg 2x daily	· Headache · Nausea · Rash	· VA-QT	· Slow heart rate · Prolonged QT interval · LVH	· CHF · CAD

mg: milligrams, **mcg**: micrograms, **hrs**: hours, **CHF**: congestive heart failure, **CAD**: coronary artery disease, **CM**: cardiomyopathy, **VHD**: valvular heart disease, **LVH**: left ventricular hypertrophy, **VA-QT**: ventricular arrhythmias due to QT prolongation, **y.o.**: years old
*Needs to be used with an AV nodal blocking agent

Table 17

of medicine when it comes to pharmaceutical therapeutics, like oncology and immune conditions where monoclonal antibodies have been major steps forward, there is no counterpart to that in arrhythmia medicine.

In large studies, antiarrhythmic drugs have a success rate of 60 percent at best. The most effective of all the drugs is amiodarone, but it has several organ toxicities. The choice of antiarrhythmic is based on underlying heart disease and kidney and liver function.

The class Ic antiarrhythmics are sodium channel blockers. These include drugs such as propafenone and flecainide. Sodium channel blocking drugs slow the electrical impulses in the heart, so they are especially useful to help convert AFib to normal rhythm, a pill-in-pocket approach. Sodium channel blocking antiarrhythmics are contraindicated if a patient has underlying coronary artery disease, congestive heart failure, or significant preexisting electrical diseases such as significant AV nodal disease or bundle branch block.

The other main class of antiarrhythmics includes class III agents. These include amiodarone, dronedarone, sotalol, and dofetilide.

Amiodarone can be used in any patient with or without heart disease. It causes multiple side effects, which increase if high doses are used for long periods of time. Four main organs are affected: liver (inflammation called hepatitis), thyroid (reduces or increases function), eyes (corneal deposits), and lungs (fibrosis, or scarring). Amiodarone can be used intravenously or orally. When the drug is started, it is usually started at a high dose then gradually tapered because it takes several weeks to reach a therapeutic level. Likewise, when the drug is stopped, it takes several weeks to clear from the body. I have a love-hate relationship with this drug; my first research paper as a medical intern was on amiodarone.

Dronedarone is similar in chemical composition to amiodarone but without the iodine molecule. Without the iodine, it has a lower incidence of toxicities but also has a lower success rate. Dronedarone is contraindicated in the setting of congestive heart failure, but can be used with underlying coronary artery disease.

Sotalol is a beta-blocker with a potassium channel blocker property. It prolongs refractoriness of the cell, which essentially means that it is more difficult for premature beats to initiate arrhythmias.

Dofetilide is a similar potassium channel blocker without the beta-blocker effect. This also means it does not have the typical side effects of beta-blockers such as fatigue, insomnia, or dizziness. Therefore, it tends to be better tolerated. With both sotalol and dofetilide, there is a rare risk of a rapid and sometimes life-threatening arrhythmia from the ventricles called *torsades de pointes*, which is related to prolongation of the QT interval on the EKG. It is for this reason that dofetilide, in particular, is started in the hospital under close telemetry monitoring.

CARDIOVERSION

Cardioversion is an outpatient noninvasive procedure by which an electrical impulse is applied to the heart to reset the rhythm. Typically, a person is deeply sedated for a few minutes. The recovery is fast, so the patient can go home within an hour or two after the procedure. Sometimes, a transesophageal echo is done before the procedure to confirm that no blood clots are present before proceeding. Acute success rate of cardioversion is dependent on duration of AFib. For AFib present less than six months,

Cardioversion

Outpatient procedure whereby a patient is deeply sedated while an electrical impulse is applied to the heart through adhesive patches on the skin (chest and back). Used to convert AFib to normal sinus rhythm.

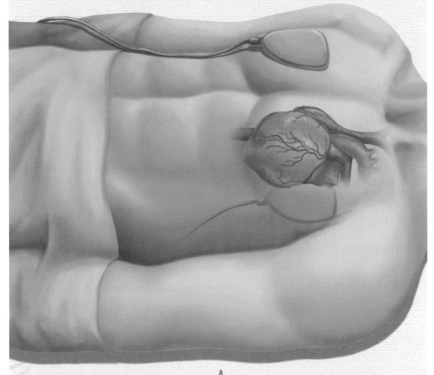

Before Cardioversion
Heart in Atrial Fibrilliation

After Cardioversion
Heart in Sinus Rhythm

Figure 18

the success rate typically is over 90 percent. AFib existing for more than one year has a success rate of less than 50 percent. In many cases, cardioversion works to restore the rhythm but AFib recurs. Cardioversion is an acute treatment—it does nothing to prevent AFib. Sometimes cardioversion is used to clarify if someone is having symptoms from AFib. If energy or well-being improves with conversion to normal rhythm, then these are the AFib symptoms a patient has. That way, if AFib recurs, there is justification to go to the next step in treatment—medication or ablation.

DEVICES

As electrophysiologists, we have traditionally told people that pacemakers are not used to treat AFib. They are used to treat problems with slow heartbeats (bradycardia). However, a pacemaker can be used in certain scenarios related to AFib. In some cases, if someone needs to be on medication to maintain sinus rhythm, and that medication slows the heartbeat too much, then a pacemaker can be implanted to safely allow the use of medication.

This is most common in patients with tachycardia-bradycardia syndrome and sick sinus syndrome. A second way pacemakers can be used for atrial fibrillation is an algorithm that suppresses the premature atrial contractions that trigger AFib. One company has an algorithm that detects the underlying heartbeat, and if enough premature beats are seen, it will pace the atrium five to ten beats faster to suppress the extra beats. In some cases, pacing at a higher heart rate can also trigger AFib (by shortening the atrial refractory period), so the data regarding these atrial fibrillation suppression algorithms are equivocal as far as benefit is concerned. Another way a pacemaker can be used to maintain normal rhythm is through antitachycardia pacing. This technology will deliver rapid atrial pacing to help stop certain types of atrial arrhythmias.

One, in particular, is atrial flutter. Atrial flutter is a rapid heart rate in the top chambers that usually goes about 300 beats per minute and is similar in some ways to atrial fibrillation. By pacing faster than the rate of the atrial flutter circuit, the impulse can block in both directions around the circuit. Remember the earlier analogy of atrial flutter being like a runner on a racetrack with the racetrack being the arrhythmia circuit? Antitachycardia pacing for atrial flutter is like a faster runner setting down hurdles for the slower runner to stop. After the hurdles are set, the faster runner also stops so that a normal rhythm can resume. A person does not typically feel anything when the algorithm applies. Data shows that when this algorithm is applied, there is a reduction in the number of atrial flutter and atrial fibrillation episodes, and in the duration of those episodes.

The above discussion of pacemakers primarily focuses on dual-chamber pacemakers, which means there is one pacemaker lead in the atrium and one in the ventricle. This is because the atria and ventricles need to be synchronized with each other to maintain a normal cardiac chamber contraction sequence. To this end, these devices are typically implanted via the left or right subclavian vein, with the left more commonly used. It is located underneath the clavicle (collarbone).

A different use of pacemakers, for AFib, is in the form of rate control (AV node ablation and pacemaker). Here, only the right ventricle needs to be paced because usually these patients are in

Single-Chamber Pacemaker

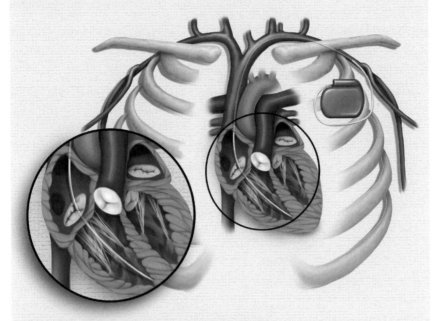

Dual-Chamber Pacemaker

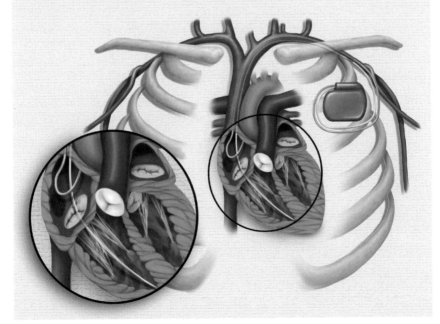

Figure 19

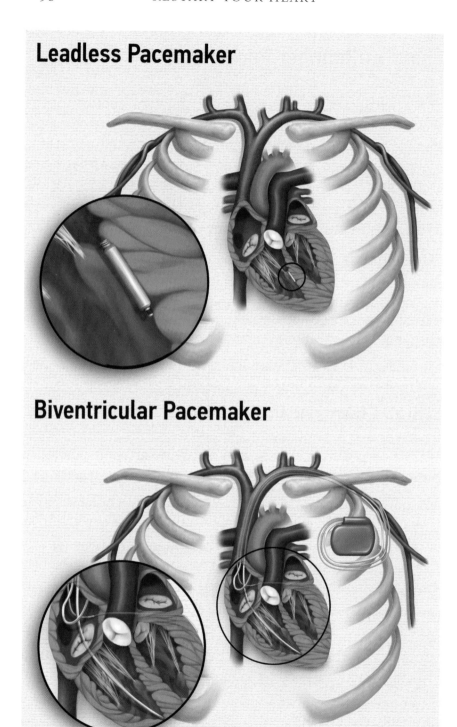

Leadless Pacemaker

Biventricular Pacemaker

Figure 20

permanent AFib, and the purpose of the pacemaker is to support the slow heartbeat that results from ablating the AV node. In recent years, another option for pacing the right ventricle has been developed, called leadless pacing. Here, rather than a pacemaker lead being placed within the subclavian vein and entering into the heart, there is a pellet-like device that is placed via the femoral vein, which adheres to the heart muscle using nitinol tines (soft "hooks").

Leadless pacemakers have several advantages over traditional transvenous pacemakers. Because there are no leads, one does not have to be concerned about the fracture of the lead or wearing down of the insulation around the lead—two reasons transvenous pacemakers may need revision or removal. Because there is no needle puncture of the subclavian vein, there is no risk of lung puncture (pneumothorax). Lastly, because there is no pacemaker pocket under the skin, there is no risk for bleeding or infection in that area of the body (when a pacemaker infection occurs, it usually starts in the pocket). A final advantage of leadless pacemakers is patient acceptance. Because there is no visible pacemaker under the skin, patients are not reminded every day they have an artificial device in their heart. The risks with leadless pacemakers include migration of the device, puncture of the heart muscle, and damage to the femoral blood vessel. Fortunately, these complications do not occur often. In fact, studies have shown that the complication rate with leadless pacemakers is less than with transvenous pacemakers.

Again, as a reminder, current leadless pacemakers only sense and pace in the right ventricle, so there is no synchronization with the atria. Therefore, they are most commonly used in those with permanent AFib.

ABLATION

It is important to distinguish between two types of ablation in the setting of AFib: AV node ablation versus left atrial ablation.

AV Node Ablation

AV node ablation focuses on rate control, not rhythm control. The atria remain in AFib and, therefore, almost all patients will require some form of lifelong anticoagulation (blood thinner to prevent stroke) or left atrial appendage occlusion device (discussed later). The only exceptions are those patients with a contraindication to blood thinners, who have a significant recent bleeding history, among other factors, or who cannot undergo a left atrial appendage occlusion procedure. With AV node ablation, the central electrical system, called the AV node, is ablated, which results in the heart rate slowing down significantly to the point that a pacemaker is required to support the heartbeat.

Often these patients are "pacemaker dependent," which means that if the pacemaker were to malfunction or the battery becomes depleted, the heartbeat would be slow or nonexistent to the point of causing fainting without warning and resulting in trauma or even death. That being said, with current-day pacemaker technology and remote monitoring of devices, the likelihood of either occurrence is relatively low. This type of ablation is "irreversible" in that the AV node cells typically do not grow back to restore the heartbeat. AV node ablation was performed much more often

AV Node Ablation

Radiofrequency energy is applied to the AV node to slow the heart rate. Typically used in combination with a pacemaker for patients in permanent AFib, where the heart rate cannot be adequately controlled with medication. Outpatient procedure that is typically 1-2 hours in duration.

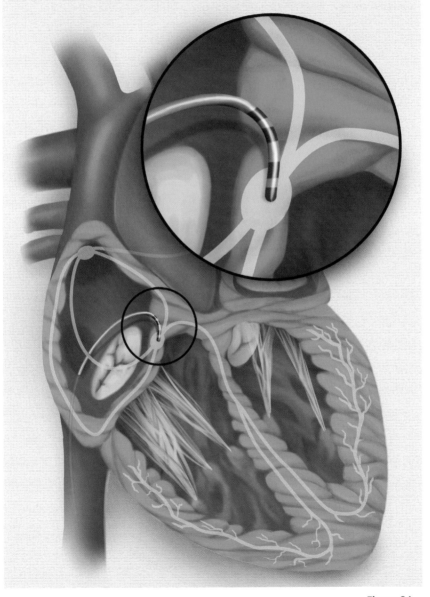

Figure 21

in the past, when left atrial ablation had lower success rates and higher risk. That ratio has changed over the years to favor left atrial ablation in more patients than AV node ablation.

Usually, AV node ablation is performed in patients who have permanent AFib, in which the rhythm cannot be restored to sinus, or the risk of left atrial ablation exceeds the likelihood of sinus rhythm. Generally, this type of ablation is performed in older patients. A significant benefit of this type of ablation is the ability to often eliminate drugs used for rate control, such as beta-blockers, calcium channel blockers, or digoxin.

As we age, the incidence of medication side effects and drug-drug interactions increases, so eliminating any medication is desirable. Another attractive aspect of the pacemaker component of AV node ablation is the advent of leadless pacemakers. As mentioned, current leadless pacemakers detect signals and pace in the right ventricle only. Therefore, they can be used in permanent AFib where synchronization of the atria and ventricles is not needed, as it would be in normal sinus rhythm.

Left Atrial Ablation

Catheter ablation of atrial fibrillation has been around since the mid-1990s. It was pioneered by the French electrophysiologist Michel Haïssaguerre. The first publication regarding this was in the September 1998 issue of the *New England Journal of Medicine*. Here, patients with paroxysmal atrial fibrillation (PAF) were studied. They underwent electrophysiology studies whereby catheters were inserted in different parts of the electrical system. In many patients, it was found that premature atrial beats, which triggered

AFib, originated from the pulmonary veins. This formed the foundation of AFib ablation: pulmonary vein isolation.

Normally, veins and arteries do not have electrical tissue. In the case of the pulmonary veins, there are muscular sleeves that reach from the left atrial tissue into the pulmonary veins. These sleeves contain cells with spontaneous electrical activity (automaticity and triggered), as well as short circuits (reentry). The principle behind AFib ablation is isolating the pulmonary veins from the rest of the heart so they cannot trigger AFib, which is why the procedure is called pulmonary vein isolation. As an aside, it is interesting to note that the cells within the pulmonary veins are similar to the cells in the left atrium chamber proper, as they share a similar embryological origin.

Over the years, multiple iterations of ablation techniques and developments in technology have led to modern-day AFib ablation that can be accomplished within two hours and is entirely outpatient. Catheters are placed in the femoral veins, which lead to the right side of the heart. A transseptal catheterization is performed to allow catheters to go from the right atrium to the left atrium under direct ultrasound guidance. The initial part of the procedure is 3-D electroanatomic mapping. Here, a color-coding algorithm identifies the abnormal and normal regions, ablation is performed, and the area is remapped to confirm electrical isolation of the veins.

There are two endpoints to the procedure: the elimination of pulmonary vein potentials (the abnormal electrical signatures for AFib cells) and noninducibility of atrial fibrillation with rapid atrial pacing and IV isoproterenol (adrenaline) and/or adenosine.

TYPES OF 3-D MAPPING CATHETERS

Multiple electrodes create color-coded maps of signals

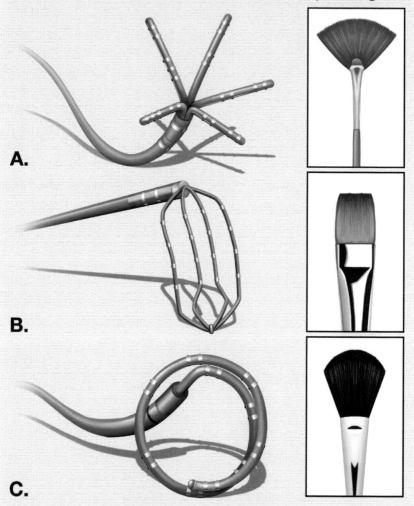

A.

B.

C.

There are a variety of three-dimensional mapping catheters, which use algorithms to translate electrical information into color, in order to guide localization of abnormal circuits and measure successful endpoints after ablation. The catheters have multiple small electrodes to rapidly collect information in large "brushstrokes." This is similar to a paintbrush concept.

Figure 22a

3-D Mapping during AFib Ablation

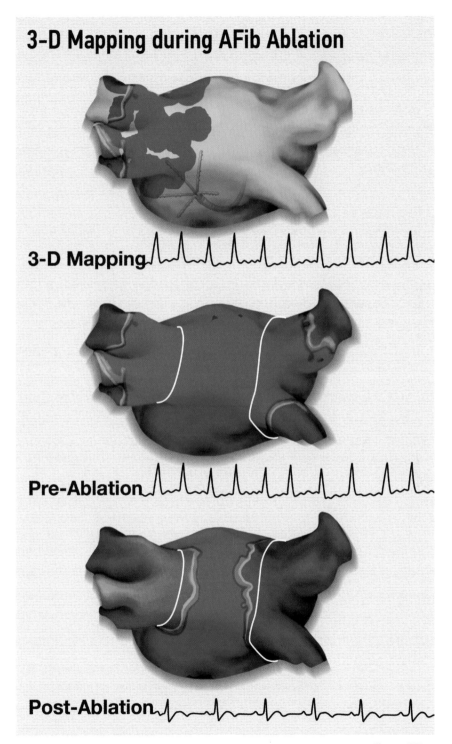

3-D Mapping

Pre-Ablation

Post-Ablation

Figure 22b

From a pre-op standpoint, not much is required. It starts with basic blood work. Then, often a 3-D computed tomography (CT) is done to anatomically characterize the pulmonary veins as a road map, as well as exclude any clots in the left atrium or appendage. It is known that AFib can recur in up to 15 percent to 20 percent of paroxysmal AFib patients who undergo pulmonary vein isolation.

There are two reasons for recurrent AFib: "reconnection" of the muscular sleeves due to nontransmural lesion, and other extrapulmonary vein foci, which include the superior vena cava, ligament of Marshall, coronary sinus, left atrial appendage, and posterior wall. Sometimes these foci are not apparent at the original procedure because the pulmonary vein triggers suppress them. Regarding reconnection and nontransmural lesion, the advent of contact force-sensing catheters has reduced that significantly. Deflectable sheaths have also helped.

In this procedure, two main technologies are used: radiofrequency contact force-sensing (RF) and cryoballoon. Other energy sources such as laser, microwave, and ultrasound have been studied and used with varying success rates but often with additional risks. A large study, the FIRE and ICE Trial, showed equivalent outcome of freedom from AFib, in both cryo and RF. There are a few ways these technologies differed in the trial. All differences were statistically significant.

Normally, radiation in the form of X-ray is required for ablation to guide catheters in the heart. With RF, not much X-ray is typically required. More is required for cryo (statistically significant). The procedure time for RF was longer than with cryo. Lastly, cryo requires the use of IV contrast to image the

Cryoballoon Ablation

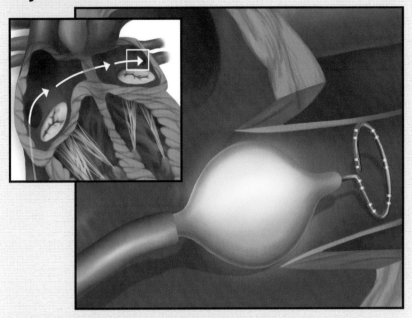

Radiofrequency Ablation

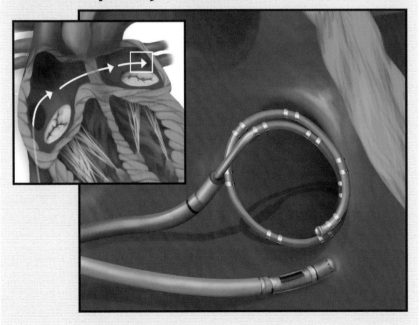

Figure 23

pulmonary veins and RF does not. The idea behind RF is that energy stirs up the molecules in the tissue, which creates thermal energy that destroys tissue. In the case of cryo, this freezes, injures, then destroys the tissue. Phrenic nerve injury is more common with cryo. So phrenic nerve pacing is performed during right pulmonary vein ablation. RF requires one access point (right femoral vein), and cryo requires two (right and left femoral), due to the fact that the cryo catheter is large enough that it should be used alone on one side.

Remote magnetic navigation is a robotic ablation technology that also can be used to treat AFib. Here, two large magnets rotate around a patient and are driven by a combination of computer mouse movements and clicks that direct a magnetic field to "pull" the catheter through the heart, as the catheter has magnets at the tip. Advantages include continuous contact with tissue despite the patient breathing and their heart beating, increased safety, increased accuracy, and reduced X-ray exposure for patient and physician. The safety aspect is due to the catheter being ultra-soft at the tip. This technology has two primary limitations: There is no discrete way to measure the amount of force being applied by the catheter to the tissue surface, and the cost of the technology is prohibitive for many medical centers.

With regard to persistent AFib ablation, additional lesions may be performed. Sometimes this involves creating lines of ablation that act as "fences" to contain the abnormal impulses. These additional lesion sets can include left atrial posterior wall isolation (PWI), left atrial roof line, right atrial cavo-tricuspid isthmus (CTI) flutter line, and complex fractionated atrial electrogram

Robotic Catheter Ablation

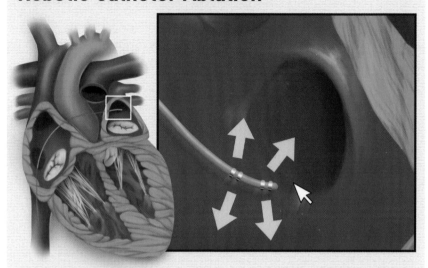

Robotic ablation technology uses an external magnetic field to direct an ablation catheter, which has magnets near the tip. The magnetic field is controlled via a computer mouse interface. Accuracy and precision is within 1 mm. Catheter is ultra soft, which increases safety. Rather than pushing a manual ablation catheter, the catheter is pulled through the heart.

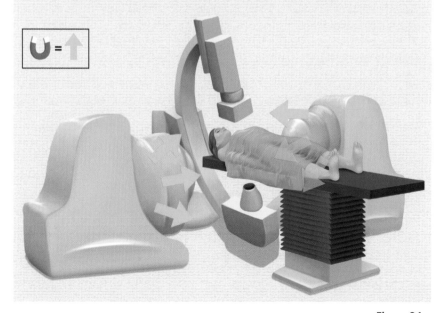

Figure 24

Convergent AFib Ablation

Pre-Ablation

Pre-ablation 3-D electrical map of left atrial posterior wall and pulmonary veins. Green and yellow intermixed with red indicates abnormal electrical tissue, which can trigger and sustain AFib.

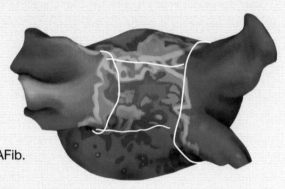

Convergent Ablation

Convergent ablation catheter creates linear lesions along the left atrial posterior wall and posterior part of the pulmonary veins. Catheter is inserted through a small incision just inferior to the sternum. A fiberoptic scope helps guide positioning.

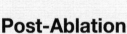

Post-Ablation

Post-ablation 3-D mapping after epicardial and endocardial ablation shows uniform red along the posterior wall and pulmonary veins. This indicates successful elimination of abnormal electrical tissue termed isolation.

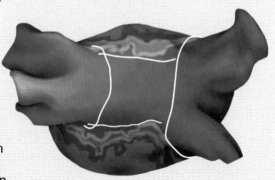

Figure 25

ablation (CFAE). The goal of persistent AFib ablation is to limit the ability of the heart to sustain AFib, the fire. This is in contrast to paroxysmal atrial fibrillation, where the goal is to eliminate triggers, the sparks. For persistent AFib and long-standing persistent AFib, hybrid ablation using an endocardial (inside of heart) approach and epicardial (outside of heart) approach can be very effective. A newer technique called the Convergent Procedure utilizes a minimally invasive approach.

AFib can initially occur after ablation. This is because it takes time for the lesions to scar and connect with one another to create a solid line of electrical insulation from abnormal impulses. During this time, impulses can "get through." Pulmonary vein isolation is like building a wall around a castle. The mortar between bricks needs time to solidify. Similarly, linear lines are like creating fences, which contain disorganized cattle.

Certain types of arrhythmias can occur as a result of gaps in lines or new, diseased tissue. These include post-ablation atrial tachycardia and atypical atrial flutter. These are known as post-ablation atrial arrhythmias.

The relationship between scarring, AFib, and success rates deserves special attention. The University of Utah has pioneered research in this area. Investigators performed special cardiac MRI scans, which have the ability to measure the amount of scar tissue in the left atrial chamber (scar burden). They discovered that some patients with paroxysmal AFib, who normally are thought of as early in the disease process, may in some cases have a large amount of scar tissue. Similarly, they found that some patients with persistent AFib, which is a more advanced form of the disease, had less scar tissue than expected. Moreover, the researchers found that the greater the scar burden, the greater the recurrence rate after any therapeutic intervention.

Finally, recent data demonstrates a lower incidence of Alzheimer's and other types of dementia in patients who have undergone atrial fibrillation ablation in an attempt to maintain sinus rhythm. The field of electrophysiology will continue to investigate this intriguing finding.

For additional information about ablation, please see "Frequently Asked Questions about Ablation" at the end of this chapter.

Rate Control

The previous discussion was about ways in which sinus rhythm can be maintained (rhythm control). Another strategy for overcoming AFib is rate control. In patients where sinus rhythm cannot be maintained due to the chronicity of the disease and progressive scarring of the electrical system, controlling the heart rate affords the ability to prevent congestive heart failure, ameliorate symptoms, and prevent hospitalization. Two treatment strategies are used for rate control: (1) medication, and (2) AV node ablation plus pacemaker. We will first review medication options, then discuss AV node ablation and pacemaker.

Beta-blockers work as adrenaline modifiers. We know that elevated adrenaline can act as a trigger for AFib, as well as for premature atrial beats that can trigger AFib. Since elevated adrenaline raises the heart rate, it is not surprising that a primary effect of beta-blockers is to lower the heart rate. Beta-blockers have a 20 percent to 30 percent success rate overall in maintaining sinus rhythm. However, they can be very effective in controlling the

Rate Control Drugs

Class	Drug	Dose	Side effects	Serious reactions	Avoid use in	Can be used with
II (beta-blocker)	Metoprolol (Toprol, Lopressor)	25-100mg 2x daily for short acting (tartrate) and 1x daily for long acting (succinate)	· Fatigue · Dizziness			· CAD · LVH · Liver disease · CHF (compensated)
	Atenolol (Tenormin)	25-100mg 1x daily	· Sleep disturbance (vivid dreams, insomnia) · Depression		· Depression	· CAD · LVH · Liver disease
	Carvedilol (Coreg)	3.125-35mg 2x daily for short acting and 20-80mg 1x daily for long acting	· Erectile dysfunction · Hair loss · Aggravation of asthma and wheezing	· CHF exacerbation · Heart block · Severe low BP	· COPD/asthma · Decompensated heart failure · Decompensated CHF	· CAD · LVH · Liver disease · CHF (compensated)
	Propranolol (Inderal)	10-30mg 3-4x daily for short acting and 60-160mg 1x daily for long acting	· Shortness of breath		· Slow heart rate	· CAD · LVH · Liver disease · Anxiety
	Nebivolol (Bystolic)	2.5-10mg 1x daily	· Same as other beta-blockers but with a lower incidence of side effects			· CAD · LVH · Liver disease
Cardiac glycosides	Digoxin	0.125mg, 0.25mg	· Nausea	· Heart block · Digoxin toxicity syndrome	· Advanced kidney disease · Slow heart rate · Elderly patients	· CHF · CAD · VHD
Calcium channel blockers	Diltiazem	Immediate release: 80-120mg 2x daily Sustained release: 180-480mg 1x daily	· Cause less fatigue · No effect on erectile function · No effect on sleep · Does not aggravate asthma · Significant constipation · Ankle swelling (edema)	· Heart block · Severe drop in blood pressure	· Slow heart rate · Low blood pressure · CHF	· CAD · Kidney disease · Liver disease
	Verapamil	Immediate release: 30-90mg 3-4x daily Sustained release: 120-480mg 1x daily				

mg: milligrams, mcg: micrograms, hrs: hours, CHF: congestive heart failure, CAD: coronary artery disease, CM: cardiomyopathy, VHD: valvular heart disease, LVH: left ventricular hypertrophy, VA-QT: ventricular arrhythmias due to QT prolongation, y.o.: years old

Table 26

heart rate if someone is in atrial fibrillation. Side effects include fatigue, shortness of breath, dizziness due to lowering of blood pressure and heart rate, sleep disturbance such as vivid dreams or insomnia, erectile dysfunction, depression, and aggravation of asthma. Common beta-blockers include metoprolol, atenolol, and carvedilol.

A newer-generation beta-blocker, nebivolol (Bystolic) is reported to have a lower incidence of side effects. Another beta-blocker, propranolol, can help with anxiety symptoms associated with AFib, as well as the heart rate itself. This is because it crosses the blood-brain barrier. It is also useful in migraine prevention. Calcium channel blockers work to modify adrenaline's effect on the heart's electrical system. Like beta-blockers, they slow heart rate and lower blood pressure. They cause less fatigue, have no effect on erectile function or sleep, and do not aggravate asthma. However, they can cause significant constipation and ankle swelling (edema). Examples include diltiazem and verapamil.

Lastly, digoxin is an old drug that helps control the heart rate in AFib through its effect on the sodium/potassium channel and parasympathetic nervous system. It is especially useful if someone also has congestive heart failure due to reduced ejection fraction because it can increase the contractile function of the heart. (Ejection fraction is a measure of how well the heart muscle can contract.) A major limitation with digoxin is its narrow therapeutic index—meaning that the difference between therapeutic benefit and toxicity is small. This risk increases with age. A benefit of digoxin is that it does not lower the blood pressure, if that is a limiting factor.

An alternative to medication—or if medication is ineffective or not tolerated—is a procedure called AV node ablation and pacemaker implant. The AV node is the central portion of the heart's electrical system, which connects the atria and the ventricles. If radiofrequency ablation of the AV node is performed, the heart rate slows significantly to the point that it often cannot support the blood pressure. For this reason, a pacemaker is implanted at the time of the procedure to regulate the heartbeat. A major limitation of this approach is that it is permanent, and the patient is dependent on the pacemaker for all heartbeats. If the pacemaker were to malfunction, sudden death can result. However, the likelihood of this is very low.

Some patients require a biventricular pacemaker (paces right and left ventricles). Here there are two leads to pace the ventricles so there is a "backup," so to speak. The atria may still be fibrillating and the need for a blood thinner is still there. Often, medications can still be reduced or eliminated, especially those required to control the heart rate, because the AV node ablation and pacemaker do the job. Now, there is a leadless pacemaker that is invisible on the outside, so you wouldn't even realize if you had one. How great is that?

Stroke Prevention

Stroke prevention is paramount in atrial fibrillation. Most often this is in the form of blood thinners. There are several to choose from, often determined by comorbidities (such as kidney disease), cost, and drug/diet interactions. Warfarin is still the least

Stroke Prevention: Screening

CHA_2DS_2-VAS_c is the scoring system to determine risk of stroke with AFib. HAS-BLED is the scoring system to determine risk of bleeding with blood thinners (anticoagulation). Comparing these scores can give risk-to-benefit guidance on decisions about blood thinners.

CHA_2DS_2-VAS_c Screening Factors		YES	NO
C	Do you have **congestive heart failure**?	○ (1 pt)	○ (0 pt)
H	Do you have **high blood pressure**?	○ (1 pt)	○ (0 pt)
A	Is your **age** older than 75 years old?	○ (2 pts)	○ (0 pt)
D	Do you have **diabetes**?	○ (1 pt)	○ (0 pt)
S	Have you ever had a **stroke** or do you show signs of having experienced a TIA or a mini-stroke?	○ (2 pts)	○ (0 pt)
V	Do you have **vascular disease** in your history (such as a prior heart attack, peripheral artery diease, aortic plaque)?	○ (1 pt)	○ (0 pt)
A	Is your **age** between 65 and 74 years old?	○ (1 pt)	○ (0 pt)
S	Is your **sex** female?	○ (1 pt)	○ (0 pt)
Total			

HAS-BLED Screening Factors		YES	NO
H	Do you have **hypertension**?	○ (1 pt)	○ (0 pt)
A	Do you have **abnormal kidney or liver function**?	○ (1-2 pts)	○ (0 pt)
S	Have you had a **stroke**?	○ (1 pt)	○ (0 pt)
B	Do you have a prior history of **bleeding** issues?	○ (1 pt)	○ (0 pt)
L	**Labile** INRs?	○ (1 pt)	○ (0 pt)
E	Are you **elderly** (over 65)?	○ (1 pt)	○ (0 pt)
D	Do you take **drugs**: specifically, anitplatelets, NSAIDs, or abuse alcohol?	○ (1-2 pts)	○ (0 pt)
Total			

Figure 27

expensive but requires blood monitoring and watching for interactions with diet and other meds. Several direct oral anticoagulants are available—rivaroxaban, apixaban, dabigatran, and edoxaban. Previously, there was not a reversal agent for these drugs in case of bleeding or need for surgery—but now there is. These drugs have been shown to have a lower risk of bleeding compared to warfarin. They are dosed based on kidney function, body weight, and age.

Still, there are some people who cannot take a blood thinner because of other bleeding problems. For these situations, three options are currently available, which fall under the category of left atrial appendage occlusion. The left atrial appendage is an anatomic structure that accounts for the majority of strokes related to AFib. Procedures can be carried out to eliminate the ability of a clot to travel from this site to the brain. These include Watchman, Lariat, and left atrial appendage ligation or removal via surgery. The hybrid ablation Convergent Procedure often has left atrial appendage clipping, called AtriClip, as an option.

It is interesting to note that atrial fibrillation is associated with many downstream problems that can be lessened by maintaining sinus rhythm, especially through ablation. These include hospitalization, heart failure, and even dementia, including Alzheimer's.

Stroke Prevention: Treatments

	Drug	Dose	Comments
Blood thinners	Apixaban (Eliquis)	2.5mg 2x daily, 5mg 2x daily	· Can be used in any kidney disease including dialysis patients · Reversal agent - Andexanet (Andexxa)
	Dabigatran (Pradaxa)	75mg 2x daily, 150mg 2x daily	· First direct acting oral anticoagulant · Reversal agent - Idarucizumab (Praxbind)
	Edoxaban (Savaysa)	30mg 1x daily, 60mg 1x daily	· Do not use if CrCL > 95 mL/min (supernormal kidney function) · Reversal agent - Andexanet (Andexxa)
	Rivaroxaban (Xarelto)	15mg 1x daily, 20mg 1x daily	· Reversal agent - Andexanet (Andexxa)
	Warfarin (Coumadin)	Varies to achieve target INR 2.0-3.0	· Longest studied blood thinner · Reversal agents - vitamin K and FFP

	Device	Visual
Procedures	Lariat	
	Watchman	
	Atri-Clip	

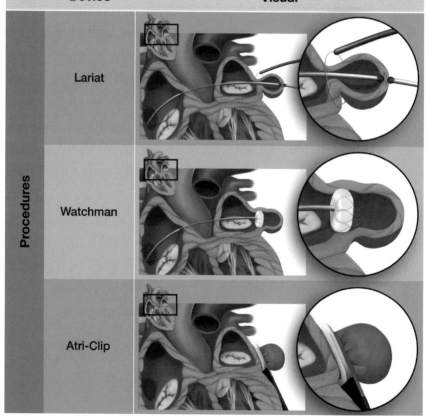

Figure 28

Action Plan

1. Learn about AFib: Study this book, look up information on trusted medical websites (getsmartaboutafib.com, stopafib. org). You can jot down ideas and points to remember in the **Notes** section of this book.

2. Complete the Self-Assessment - AFib Risk Factors list in one sitting and commit to at least two of the twenty-one-day goals. Share these with a friend or loved one so you have an accountability partner.

3. Complete the Self-Assessment - AFib Triggers list in one sitting and commit to at least two of the twenty-one-day goals. See your primary care physician to discuss these two goals so you have an accountability partner.

Frequently Asked Questions about Drugs

What are the different types of rate-control drugs?

Rate-control drugs slow the pulse rate in the setting of AFib. These drugs are not specifically designed to stop AFib episodes or terminate an episode. That being said, they sometimes can do so by reducing the number of premature beats that may trigger AFib and by reducing the circulating levels of adrenaline—beta-blockers, in particular—that spike during AFib and help to perpetuate it. The two most common classes are the beta-adrenergic blocker agents and the calcium channel blocker agents. The oldest beta-blocker is atenolol, which is dosed once a day typically. Metoprolol is another common one used.

There is immediate-acting metoprolol called metoprolol tartrate, which is dosed two to three times per day, and there is sustained-release metoprolol called metoprolol succinate that is dosed once a day. The rate-limiting factor with this drug is getting insurance coverage by certain payers.

For calcium channel blockers, the two most commonly used are diltiazem and verapamil. These come in immediate-release forms (dosed three to four times per day) and sustained release (dosed one to two times per day).

What are the side effects of rate-control drugs?

Beta-blockers can cause low heart rate, low blood pressure, dizziness, fainting, fatigue, and shortness of breath. They also can aggravate asthma, cause insomnia or vivid dreams, exacerbate depression, exacerbate erectile dysfunction, or impair blood sugar. Calcium channel blockers can cause low heart rate, low blood pressure, dizziness, fainting, fatigue (usually not to the degree of beta-blockers), constipation, and ankle swelling (edema).

What are the different types of rhythm-control or antiarrhythmic drugs?

There are two main classes: sodium channel blockers (class I) and potassium channel blockers (class III). The sodium channel blockers most commonly used are propafenone and flecainide. They should be used only when significant structural heart disease (coronary artery disease, heart surgery, heart failure) has been ruled out. Propafenone has immediate-acting and sustained-release formulations. The immediate-acting comes as 150 mg and 225 mg tabs usually dosed three times a day. The sustained-release form comes as 225 mg, 325 mg, and 425 mg tabs and is usually dosed twice a day. A certain percentage of the population slowly metabolizes propafenone, making them more susceptible to the heart-rate-slowing effects in particular. Flecainide is typically dosed twice a day. It comes as 50 mg, 100 mg, and 150 mg tablets, with the maximum daily dose being around 300 mg. Both propafenone and flecainide are more potent at faster heart rates, which is why they are sometimes used to terminate an AFib episode with a pill-in-the-pocket approach.

Less commonly used class I agents include disopyramide, procainamide, and quinidine. Disopyramide seems to have a specific benefit in those patients whose AFib is triggered through the parasympathetic nervous system (vagus nerve). It comes in immediate-release and sustained-release formulations. Procainamide and quinidine are rarely used today due to a high side effect profile.

The class III agents include sotalol, dronedarone, amiodarone, and dofetilide. Sotalol has beta-blocker and potassium channel blocking properties. Dronedarone is similar in chemical composition to amiodarone but without the iodine molecule. Iodine is important in thyroid hormone metabolism, and it can cause amiodarone to affect the liver, lungs, and thyroid. By removing iodine, dronedarone does not have that side effect profile but it is also less effective. It is thought that the iodine modification, which occurs with amiodarone, may be partly antiarrhythmic because of its effect on thyroid metabolism.

Both classes of drugs affect certain EKG intervals that can increase the risk of causing abnormal rhythms (proarrhythmia). There are certain risk factors for proarrhythmia, which include baseline prolonged EKG intervals (PR, QRS, QTc), the presence of structural heart disease, abnormal kidney or liver function, and advanced age. Flecainide and propafenone should not be used with patients with structural heart disease (prior heart attack, coronary artery disease, congestive heart failure, etc.), significant AV block or sick sinus syndrome, or prolonged QRS or QTc intervals.

What are the side effects of antiarrhythmic drugs?

Flecainide can cause headaches; propafenone can cause fatigue, dizziness, low heart rate, and a metallic taste in the mouth. Amiodarone can cause lung fibrosis, liver inflammation, over- or underactive thyroid function, skin photosensitivity, and corneal eye deposits. With amiodarone, typically lung function, liver function, thyroid function, and eye health are assessed each year. Dronedarone can cause gastrointestinal upset. Sotalol can cause fatigue, low heart rate, and dizziness, exacerbate asthma, and produce other side effects typical of beta-blocker medication. Dofetilide can cause headaches. Sotalol and dofetilide can predispose to *torsades de pointes* ventricular tachycardia, which is a proarrhythmia related to prolongation of the QT interval on the EKG. Dofetilide and sotalol are usually started in the hospital, under careful cardiac monitoring for arrhythmias, due to the risk of QT prolongation.

How is a drug chosen to use for treatment?

The biggest challenge with drug therapy for AFib is that all of them can affect both the ventricles and the atria. That means that drugs can cause abnormal heart rhythms, some of which can be very dangerous. This is called proarrhythmia. So, the choice of drug is based on which clinical factors a patient may or may not have that would increase the risk for specific side effects and toxicities. For example, the class Ic drugs like flecainide and propafenone must be avoided in patients with structural heart disease (prior heart attack, congestive heart failure, etc.), because they can increase mortality in those patients. Dronedarone needs to be avoided in congestive heart failure because it can increase mortality. Amiodarone should be avoided, if possible, in patients with advanced lung disease, due to its potential for toxicity.

How do drugs compare to other treatments for AFib?

For acute conversion of AFib of recent onset to normal rhythm, electrical cardioversion is superior to chemical conversion. Chemical conversion can be done with oral flecainide or propafenone, or IV ibutilide, which is a potassium channel blocker similar to oral dofetilide. For long-term maintenance of sinus rhythm, it is now well established that drug therapy is at best 60 percent effective. This is with the most powerful of all the drugs, amiodarone, which also has multiple side effects. Other drugs have even less efficacy. Ablation has a success rate as high as 85 percent to 90 percent in paroxysmal AFib patients and can be as high as 70 percent to 80 percent in persistent AFib. Pacemakers are not specifically used to treat AFib, but can benefit patients.

Frequently Asked Questions about Devices

What is a pacemaker?

A pacemaker is an implantable cardiac device that is primarily used for symptoms related to a slow heartbeat. Pacemakers have other features that may be useful in managing associated conditions such as atrial fibrillation. The pacemaker is composed of two parts: the pulse generator, often referred to as the "battery," and the leads (wires). The pulse generator is actually more than just a housing for the battery. It also acts as the "brain" of the system, having circuitry and algorithms, which ensure proper device function.

A pacemaker "battery change" involves removing the old pulse generator and implanting a new one. For the patient, this is functionally like having a brand-new pacemaker. The leads typically stay in place because scar tissue forms on them over time. If they need to be removed due to malfunction or infection, this can be done by using an extraction system. The extraction system typically consists of different tools including a laser, which cuts through the scar tissue. There are four types of commercially available pacemakers: single-chamber transvenous, dual-chamber transvenous, biventricular transvenous (three-chamber), and leadless (not transvenous). Transvenous means that the pacemaker leads are inserted via the subclavian vein under the collarbone (clavicle).

From the subclavian vein, there is a (usually) straight shot to the superior vena cava vein, which then empties into the right atrium and right ventricle. Single-chamber means that there is one lead that is in the right ventricle. Dual-chamber means there are two leads—one in the right atrium and one in the right ventricle. Biventricular means there is one lead in the right atrium and two leads in the ventricles—one for the right ventricle and one for the left ventricle. A leadless pacemaker is a device that is inserted via the femoral vein in the leg. It is deployed by a catheter and guiding sheath (tube), and there is a fixation mechanism at the tip that hooks into the heart muscle to prevent it from moving. To date, only single-chamber leadless pacemakers are available. There is ongoing work being done to develop more advanced leadless pacemakers.

Why do I need one?

The most common diagnoses for dual-chamber pacemaker implants include sick sinus syndrome, tachycardia-bradycardia syndrome, and AV block. Sick sinus syndrome means that the group of cells located in the sinus node, which set the heartbeat, have developed scarring that slows down the electrical impulses. Think of it as arthritis of the electrical system. Risk factors for the development of this scarring include age, diabetes, high blood pressure, coronary artery disease, atrial fibrillation, sleep apnea, and obesity.

The most common reasons for a single-chamber pacemaker implant are symptomatic bradycardia or AV block in a patient with permanent atrial fibrillation, or as part of an AV node ablation procedure. The advent of leadless single-chamber pacemakers has provided another option for patients who would normally undergo a single-chamber transvenous pacemaker implant.

Biventricular pacemakers are specifically used to resynchronize the timing of the right and left ventricles. Some patients with advanced congestive heart failure may develop a bundle branch block. This means there is a significant time delay between the right and left sides of the heart contracting. This results in an inefficient pump, like pistons in an engine being out of alignment. By pacing the right and left ventricles and synchronizing with the atria, the heart's pump performance can increase. Oftentimes biventricular pacemakers are used in combination with an implantable defibrillator, which paces or shocks the heart into normal rhythm if a patient is suffering from a life-threatening ventricular arrhythmia/cardiac arrest.

What does the procedure entail?

Pacemakers are outpatient, minimally invasive procedures nowadays. Some type of conscious sedation is used for most patients except those who require airway support (patients with sleep apnea) or when conscious sedation would cause unwanted reactions (elderly with dementia). In those cases, MAC or general anesthesia may be used. A local anesthetic is also injected into the area. Some physicians will perform a venogram, where an injection of contrast is done to confirm that the subclavian vein is open to allow for lead implantation.

This is especially needed if a pacemaker is being upgraded, as when a new lead is being added. Access to the venous system is either by a subclavian vein puncture, an axillary vein puncture, or a cephalic vein cutdown. The leads are placed in the heart using a tool called a stylet, which is a thin metal wire that can be shaped and torqued to position the lead in different locations.

Once a satisfactory location has been found, the lead is anchored in place with either a fixation screw on the tip or a tined tip, which hooks into the heart muscle. In most cases, a fixation screw is used. The leads are tested by a machine to make sure the "numbers" are adequate: amount of energy to make the pacemaker cause the heart to beat (capture threshold in volts), the size of the electrical signal in millivolts, and the lead impedance, which is a measure of resistance in the system. A very high impedance means the lead may not be in contact with the tissue and a very low impedance may indicate other clinical concerns. The leads are typically sutured to the pectoralis major muscle, and then the pacemaker pocket is irrigated with antibiotic solution and closed with suture and other devices (Steri-Strips, Dermabond, etc.). The procedure takes typically sixty to ninety minutes. Most patients stay overnight to make sure the lead does not move or dislodge or to be monitored for any significant bleeding.

What are the risks?

Risks include stroke, heart attack, death, bleeding, infection, pneumothorax (lung puncture), cardiac tamponade and emergency surgery (heart puncture), lead dislodgement, and subsequent device recall. The overall incidence of these risks is about 1 percent to 2 percent. The risk of major complications is fairly low contemporarily, with improvement in technique and technology.

What are my limitations after the procedure?

After the procedure, there is no heavy lifting (over ten pounds, usually) with the left arm or lifting of the left arm over the shoulder for four weeks. This is because the left arm is used most often with the procedure, because of straighter anatomy for the lead to enter the heart. Pacemakers can be implanted on the right side, as well. Driving restrictions vary from institution to institution, but definitely not within the first twenty-four to forty-eight hours following the procedure, due to the residual effects of sedation.

How often do I need to be seen for evaluation of my pacemaker?

Most pacemakers now have remote monitoring capability, which means in theory a patient needs to be seen in the office only once or twice a year. Since we often use pacemaker data to manage AFib patients, some people may be seen more frequently. If any programming changes are required, an office visit is needed. Most insurances typically cover up to four office visits per year.

How long does the battery last?

This varies a little by company and by the amount of pacing needed. On average, eight-plus years is most common. Some companies advertise a very long battery life. The idea behind prolonging battery life is to minimize the number of pacemaker generator changes in someone's lifetime, which reduces their risk of device injury and infection. One of the main goals of an office pacemaker check is to program to maximize battery life. There is typically not an arm restriction (over the shoulder) after a generator change.

Do I have any restrictions like microwaves, cell phones, airports?

Generally speaking, there are no significant interactions between devices and many electronics. The main issue is avoiding strong electromagnetic fields, such as an electrical power plant or standing over a running car motor. It is recommended to either keep a cell phone in a shirt pocket opposite to the side of the pacemaker or in a pants pocket. In airports, we advise patients to check with the local TSA protocol. Most will do a pat-down search. No wands should be used over pacemaker devices.

What company are you using and why?

In some ways, most pacemakers are similar regardless of company. That being said, there are certain features that may prompt your physician to recommend one over another. Medtronic has atrial preference pacing and atrial antitachycardia pacing, which help to prevent arrhythmias and treat arrhythmias. BIOTRONIK has CLS, which is an advanced rate-response sensor for those patients with AFib who also have chronotropic incompetence. These are just examples. Other companies include Boston Scientific and Abbott. Medtronic and Abbott have leadless devices.

Frequently Asked Questions about Ablation

What is catheter ablation of atrial fibrillation?

Ablation is a minimally invasive outpatient procedure, which involves inserting a small flexible tube into the femoral vein up to the heart. A special catheter with multiple electrodes (PentaRay) identifies the abnormal cells that trigger atrial fibrillation. Then, an ablation catheter is used to target these cells.

I heard there are different types of ablation (heat vs. freezing). How do you decide?

There are three types of ablation: (1) radiofrequency ablation with a contact force-sensing catheter, (2) cryoballoon ablation, and (3) robotic magnetic ablation. The choice of ablation is based on the type of AFib (paroxysmal vs. persistent), mechanism of atrial fibrillation (pulmonary veins, extra PV foci, substrate), size of the left atrium, associated triggering arrhythmias (atrial flutter, WPW, SVT, atrial tachycardia), associated medical conditions and overall health, technologies available at the hospital, and your doctor's experience with different technologies.

Clinical studies have shown equal efficacy between radiofrequency ablation and cryoballoon ablation.

What is actually being done in the heart with an AFib ablation?

There are four veins (pulmonary veins) in the top left chamber of the heart (left atrium), which emit erratic impulses to cause atrial fibrillation. Ablation electrically isolates the veins from triggering AFib. As an analogy, if the vein represents a wire with a breach in the insulation, catheter ablation seals the breach, thereby making the wire function normally.

Why do some people have more than one ablation? Some people (doctors, patients) say ablation does not work.

Treatment of AFib is individualized to the patient. No two patients are treated with the same techniques or technologies. Some patients respond to a single ablation. Some require multiple ablations, depending on duration of AFib, size of the left atrium, associated medical problems, and type of AFib (paroxysmal, persistent, chronic).

The most common reasons for AFib recurrence after ablation are regrowth of ablated tissue and/or development of new circuits.

Success depends on the type of AFib (paroxysmal, persistent, chronic), size of the left atrium, amount of scar tissue in the atria, optimization of contributing factors (high blood pressure, diabetes, obesity, sleep apnea, heavy alcohol use, smoking), physician experience and procedural volume, technique(s) used, and technologies available.

What is done before ablation (pre-op)?

A 3-D CT scan is done before the procedure, which acts as an anatomical road map. In certain patients, a transesophageal echo is done before the procedure. Your doctor will decide which imaging tests need to be done based on your type of atrial fibrillation and the blood thinners you may take.

What happens on the day of ablation?

The ablation is an outpatient procedure with an overnight stay for observation purposes.

The duration is approximately three hours, sometimes longer and sometimes shorter, depending on the number of circuits, which are mapped during the diagnostic portion of the procedure (it is different from person to person).

Three to four catheters are inserted in either or both femoral veins, depending on the patient's requirements. The veins are large and the catheters are small. After the procedure, the incision is the size of a razor nick and is barely noticeable.

A Foley catheter may or may not be inserted into your bladder during the procedure, while you are asleep. This is to monitor your urine output and make it easier for you to urinate while you are on bed rest after the procedure. There can be some discomfort when the catheter is removed. A medication called Pyridium can be given two hours before the catheter is removed to help. Please ask your doctor or nurse.

What happens after ablation?

You are on your feet walking within a few hours after the procedure. You can return to work in three or four days and resume regular exercise in five days.

You may experience chest discomfort or shortness of breath after the procedure, related to inflammation from the ablation lesions. This is called *pericarditis*. This is completely normal and typically lasts no more than four to five days. Your doctor may prescribe medication to help with the inflammation. Over-the-counter ibuprofen works well in many cases, but your doctor will instruct you on what to do. In some cases, the chest discomfort and shortness of breath can be more intense and require stronger medications.

It is normal to have extensive bruising at the catheter insertion sites related to the blood thinners used. This will all resolve in a few weeks. Catheters are inserted in the femoral vein and the radial artery (in the wrist, to monitor continuous blood pressure during the procedure).

Can you have atrial fibrillation after ablation?

It is normal to have palpitations and atrial fibrillation after ablation due to the healing of the ablation lesions. It does not mean the procedure did not work. This usually resolves within three months. For this reason, your doctor may have you take medication to suppress AFib during healing.

What are the success rates with atrial fibrillation ablation?

Success is determined as freedom from significant atrial fibrillation at a one-year follow-up after ablation.

Some patients may require more than one procedure if tissue grows back or new sites develop. This is not necessarily predictable in any given person.

In some cases, drug therapy is required long term, in addition to ablation, for patients with long-standing persistent or chronic atrial fibrillation.

Success rates based on the type of AFib:

- Paroxysmal: 70–80 percent for first procedure, 90 percent for second procedure

- Persistent: 60–70 percent for first procedure, 80 percent for second procedure, 90 percent for third procedure plus medication

- Long-Standing Persistent: 40–50 percent for first procedure, 60–70 percent for second procedure, 80 percent for third procedure plus medication

What are the risks of ablation?

Stroke/TIA: <2 percent; heart attack: <0.1 percent; death: <0.4 percent; major bleeding: 1 percent; left atrial-esophageal fistula: <0.11 percent; cardiac tamponade: <5 percent; pulmonary vein stenosis: <1 percent; AV block: 0.01 percent; phrenic nerve paralysis: <0.4 percent; vascular injury: <1.5 percent; pericarditis: <10 percent.

STEP 2

BE
PREPARED

CHAPTER 4

Breathe

*"When you get into your car, shut the door and
be there for just half a minute. Breathe . . . Even the
busiest person has time for 30 seconds of peace."*

—**Eckhart Tolle,** spiritual teacher

*"I started to get dizzy and perspire and was short
of breath, so I called the doctor, who said, 'Okay, here's
what's going on. There's something called AFib.'"*

—**Gene Simmons,** founding member of rock band KISS

A lot of studies show that when people are told negative
news about their health, they don't absorb most of the
information because their brains are in a state of physi-
ological chaos. The brain is literally unable to process information

rationally as blood shunts away from the prefrontal cortex (center of rational thought) to the amygdala (center of emotion). This is part of the fight-or-flight response.

When we think of the fight-or-flight response, it is important to consider the different parts. Adrenaline, a substance in the bloodstream known as a catecholamine, increases in response to a stressful stimulus. It is produced by the adrenal glands, which sit atop your kidneys. The pituitary gland in the brain has influence over the adrenal glands and there is a feedback loop that controls production of adrenaline. Some of adrenaline's effects on the body include elevation of heart rate and elevation of blood pressure. This has an evolutionary advantage by allowing us (and other animals) to have more reserves available to deal with or leave a potentially dangerous situation. Furthermore, adrenaline has a direct effect on the electrical system of the heart, and elevated levels can lead to cardiac arrhythmias including AFib. When it comes to the fight-or-flight response, the body's autonomic nervous system underlies it all. It includes the sympathetic and parasympathetic components. The sympathetic component includes some of the adrenaline cascade. The parasympathetic component, also known as the "rest and relax" response, is primarily driven by the vagus nerve. The autonomic nervous system is the part of your body that controls basic functions, such as your lungs breathing and your heart beating.

Hearing the words "You have atrial fibrillation" creates the same cascade of events described above. The first words you should tell yourself when hearing the diagnosis should be "Take a deep breath. You are not alone, and it will be okay." That is way easier said than done, I know. Saying it will be okay when you don't know it will be okay is not denial or positive thinking. It is a strategy to help your mind focus on solutions and not get hijacked by reacting to stress. You'll identify the challenge, partner with an AFib specialist, and together you'll come up with a plan to deal with it.

I'm not saying this is easy to do. After all, we are dealing with your heart. When our hearts are afflicted with disease, our minds dart from fear of our own suffering to fear of our families' suffering and worry. But a calm approach is an effective approach. When our minds are calm, we are able to think in a solution-oriented manner.

Therefore, there's an important piece of information I want to share with you. *There is a way to overcome AFib.* The reason AFib is experienced differently from person to person is that it is different from person to person. To some, overcoming AFib may mean complete elimination. To others, it may mean a reduction in frequency and duration of episodes, so they feel better overall. And to others, that may mean staying in AFib and having a good quality of life due to symptom control and stroke prevention. One treatment outcome is not necessarily better than another. That is why one must be very careful comparing experiences with other people who have AFib. Don't get me wrong; there is a lot of benefit to sharing experiences. Just be mindful that this disease is unlike any other. It requires an individualized approach. One size does not fit all. This is fundamental to keep in mind when undergoing any treatment for AFib, whether it is risk factor/trigger modification, drugs, devices, ablation, or any combination of these.

Deep, mindful breathing has been shown to improve clarity of mind in order to deal with challenges. Equally important, deep breathing has now been shown to lower blood pressure and heart rate, both of which are intimately involved in the body's autonomic nervous system. In the field of cardiac electrophysiology, we have become more aware of how the autonomic nervous system is intimately intertwined with the heart's electrical system. In particular, the parasympathetic ganglionic plexi, a group of nerve bundles, are located on the outside surface of the heart near the pulmonary veins and appear to be involved in triggering and maintaining AFib. Equally important, there is evidence that autonomic modification may represent an important treatment for AFib. We have also learned that modification of the autonomic nervous system can have an impact on cardiac arrhythmias. Therefore, deep breathing has two benefits: (1) improving clarity of mind, and (2) improving the calmness of the heart.

It seems only appropriate in a chapter about breathing to introduce the concept of mindfulness. Mindfulness can be considered the process of developing an awareness of one's internal and external world without being in a reactive posture. The term *mindfulness* was probably first defined by the founder of the Mindfulness-Based Stress Reduction program, Dr. Jon Kabat-Zinn. He defines mindfulness as the "awareness that arises through paying attention, on purpose, in the present moment, non-judgmentally . . . in the service of self-understanding and wisdom."

There has been a significant increase in mindfulness research over the last several years. Mindfulness has been shown to lower heart rate, blood pressure, and circulating stress hormone levels such as cortisol and adrenaline. Meditation has similar impacts. Nobel laureate Dr. Elizabeth Blackburn has done pioneering research on the link between meditation and cell longevity. Her work has focused on telomeres, which are structures at the end of chromosomes that shorten under periods of chronic stress, thereby leading to cell death. Dr. Blackburn and colleagues found that people who meditated had higher levels of the telomere-modifying enzyme telomerase. This translated into longer telomere length, which is critical in maintaining cellular integrity and life. Higher levels of telomerase and longer telomere length create more cellular resilience, so to speak. And this means a longer and healthier life.

From a personal standpoint, I have incorporated mindfulness into my everyday life and in the practice of medicine. I have found my procedures are less stressful and more enjoyable when I regularly practice mindfulness. Mindfulness doesn't eliminate my stress; rather, it helps me look at stressful events or experiences through a different lens, a lens that is less reactive and more balanced, calm, and rational.

The key to beginning a mindfulness practice is to realize that it is a practice. There isn't a finish line one has to cross. It is a lifelong process of becoming more aware of who you are inside, and how you are interconnected to everything and everyone around you. There are many ways to start the process. I have found the smartphone app Calm to be one of the best. There are seven-day programs to get you started and the sessions are only ten minutes a day, a small amount of time in contrast to the big picture. There is also a two-minute exercise, called Emergency Calm, that you can use during periods of heightened stress. Other well-rated apps include Headspace, Insight Timer, and Simple Habit.

A product called HeartMath (heartmath.com) is very popular for stress management. It is easy to use, and sessions are only a few minutes in length. The general concept is that there is a sensor that measures "heart rate variability," which is a reflection of your underlying fight-or-flight response and level of stress. The greater the variability, the more you are in a state of restful awareness. The less the variability, the more you are in a state of stress. This makes sense since more adrenaline is produced under states of stress, which, in turn, raises heart rate and limits fluctuation in heart rate (reduced variability). Heart rate variability is used for a variety of other physiologic prediction tools, most notably in predicting the risk of sudden death and in predicting the risk of hospitalization due to congestive heart failure.

The most important method for overcoming a disease is to face it. Don't identify with it. You are not an atrial fibrillation patient. You are a person who has atrial fibrillation. It does not define you. You have a choice on how to respond to this challenge. Overcoming atrial fibrillation begins with a mind-set. Overcoming atrial fibrillation begins when you breathe.

Action Plan

1. Take three deep breaths to switch from emotional thought to rational thought.

2. Repeat to yourself, *I am not alone.*

3. You are facing a challenge that you will overcome. Remind yourself that you are not your disease.

CHAPTER 5

Build a Toolbox

*"The expectations of life depend upon diligence;
the mechanic that would perfect his
work must first sharpen his tools."*

—**Confucius,** philosopher

*"When I got back to L.A., my doctor put me
on a blood thinner. My heart is healthy now,
and I've been working to raise awareness about AFib."*

—**Kevin Nealon,** actor and comedian

As I mentioned in the Introduction, I know what it is like to have a severe illness and also overcome it. I certainly didn't have it all figured out from day one. In fact, it took a long time for me to realize that in order to face a disease,

I needed to equip myself with tools—overcoming something is not a one-time shot. It is a mind-set, a recurring challenge, and it has its ups and downs. However, when you have a collection of tools to draw upon, you can ensure you will always have an answer for any challenge you may face. This concept of a toolbox is not one of cure, but of creating resilience. The best way to conceptualize this in the setting of AFib is to think of the brain-heart connection.

Brain

The organic brain and mind have a profound effect on cardiac arrhythmias. When I say "organic brain," I am referring to the cells, electrical connections, and physiology of the three-pound slab of gray matter in your skull. When I say "mind," I am referring to your thinking process. As I've mentioned multiple times, the autonomic nervous system is critical in triggering and modifying cardiac arrhythmias. The sympathetic nervous system fight-or-flight response and the parasympathetic nervous system with the vagus nerve are the principal characters in this narrative.

Heart

I think of the heart on two levels: (1) as an organ, and (2) as a representation of a connection to yourself and those around you. As an organ, the heart has an electrical system, a coronary blood-flow system, and a valvular system. The brain connects to the heart via the autonomic nervous system. In particular, there are neural inputs into the sinus and AV nodes (sympathetic and parasympathetic), as well as nerve inputs around the base of the pulmonary veins on the epicardial portion (the outside surface) of the heart. As a representation of connection to others, the feeling of love and acceptance is often physically localized to the chest and heart. This notice of connection is emotional, mental, and physical.

We celebrate this connection every year with Valentine's Day by giving our loved ones a gift of hearts. This year, I gave my wife a Valentine's Day gift and card. Actually, I gave her three cards and a picture inside a frame, which included maps of four geographic regions we have visited together. The maps were in the shape of hearts. The cards had hearts, as well. You, too, probably shared hearts with your loved ones.

Brain-Heart Connection

Since I've now defined the brain and heart, we can now use a model of the brain-heart connection to make a toolbox. Using the same 3-Step framework in this book, you can conceptualize eight tools to manage your atrial fibrillation. Keep in mind: This is *your* toolbox. You may find some of the tools I discuss helpful, and you may find that others do not apply to you. The most important part of this process is writing it down. By writing down the tools, you ingrain these thoughts in your neural circuits. This allows you to recall them easier and integrate them into your behavioral patterns. It forces you to be specific about what you are trying to describe.

The eight tools are as follows:

Tool #1: Mindfulness

Tool #2: Exercise

Tool #3: Nature

Tool #4: Music

Tool #5: Nutrition

Tool #6: Sleep

Tool #7: Social Support System

Tool #8: Health Care Team

Tool #1: Mindfulness

There is a lot of buzz nowadays about the concept of mindfulness. Some equate mindfulness with meditation or resilience training. Regardless of semantics, the overarching concept is the same. Becoming aware of your thoughts, your body, and the world around you each moment can help you better manage any challenge that comes your way.

I developed this tool only in the last few years. In fact, I have become so passionate about it that I began teaching it to my physician colleagues. It's amazing how three deep breaths or ten minutes of quiet meditation can impact the rest of your day. For example, when the EP lab staff calls me in to scrub on a case and I am in my office, I'll stop by my car in the parking garage on the way. I'll sit in the car, turn on my Calm app (more about that later), and do a two-minute Emergency Calm session. It's a guided meditation that focuses on breath and presence. This app reminds me to put life in perspective.

The app states, "All situations, all thoughts, and all emotions are impermanent. They have beginnings and they have endings. Everything rises and passes, rises and passes." It just takes two minutes, but I promise you, it can change the rest of your day. Once I began implementing this, both my concentration and my awareness increased dramatically. I could recall knowledge from years prior to draw on during a procedure. I had a greater perspective on the procedure. My patient on the table, the staff in the room, we were all part of a team. With mindfulness, there are many ways to start. I find the easiest is with a smartphone app like Calm or Headspace. YouTube is also a good source. There are plenty of books and websites out there, too.

This idea of mindfulness in helping with cardiac arrhythmias is very interesting. There is little published in the literature regarding this. Other integrative health modalities, though, have been studied. One respected study showed that acupuncture is effective in decreasing AFib recurrences after electrical cardioversion for persistent AFib. In another study, Dr. Roberto Novoa and colleagues showed that therapeutic hypnosis was found to be associated with a statistically significant lower incidence of AFib and antiarrhythmic drug use.

Tool #2: Exercise

Exercise does several things as part of this toolbox for atrial fibrillation. Regular aerobic exercise keeps your autonomic nervous system in check, balances out adrenaline and stress hormone levels, and releases endorphins that reduce mental and emotional stress.

Aside from the rare case of exercise-induced atrial fibrillation, most of the time raising the heart rate with exercise actually suppresses the premature atrial contractions that trigger AFib.

We mentioned that very low resting heart rates in conditioned athletes may be a trigger for AFib via the vagus nerve. We really don't know how to prevent this or counsel people on it. My best recommendation is to listen to your body. I have one high-endurance athlete who goes into atrial tachycardia around 190 beats per minute every time he hits a certain threshold heart rate when he cycles. I ablated him, but part of the circuit was near the phrenic nerve that innervates the diaphragm muscle for breathing, so all the cells could not be eliminated. Here, I recommended that he lessen his cycling to remain below that triggered rate. Most of the time with AFib, this does not occur, but if it does, precautionary methods must be taken.

It is important to note that there is growing interest in studying the effects of integrative health practices on arrhythmias. In particular, a study from Dr. Dhanunjaya Lakkireddy and colleagues published in the *Journal of the American College of Cardiology* in 2013 showed that twice-weekly, sixty-minute yoga classes reduced symptomatic episodes of AFib, lowered heart rate and blood pressure, and improved quality of life in a statistically significant fashion. The heart rhythm was assessed using an event monitor and symptom diary. Symptomatic AFib episodes, symptomatic non-AFib episodes (symptoms in the absence of cardiac arrhythmia), and asymptomatic AFib episodes all showed a reduction in the yoga intervention group. This study included both control and experiment groups, as well as a three-month, noninterventional observation period followed by the three-month yoga intervention period. The authors concluded that—perhaps—yoga might reduce the neurohormonal response to triggers of stress and the fight-or-flight response.

Tool #3: Nature

It is clear that being outside in nature has a calming effect on the mind and body. Exercise can take the form of a brisk walk in the woods or around a lake. You can also choose between a strenuous or a less strenuous hike. The power of the sun in improving mood cannot be overestimated. Exposure to sunlight is thought to increase your brain's production of the neurohormone serotonin. Serotonin is associated with boosting mood and helping a person feel calm and focused. Of course, there is also the important health benefit of sunlight boosting your vitamin D production for strong bones.

When your feet touch the ground, it physically and mentally grounds you. This has been observed for centuries in various Eastern spiritual and medical traditions. Research from the University of Michigan by Marc Berman and colleagues has found time spent in the woods of the forest increases memory. It is very healing to find the beauty in your immediate environment whenever possible. This means whether you are surrounded by skyscrapers or pine trees, you are immediately aware of the hidden beauty around you. The light that peeks under the curtain in the early morning dawn. The chorus shifts of birds chirping as seasons change. This is the beauty around us.

Tool #4: Music

This particular tool is near and dear to my heart. As a guitar player and singer, I find music is something readily accessible to me for stress relief or to work through a particular challenge. It is well known that music reduces anxiety for patients in a hospital. When I walk into our electrophysiology lab to scrub for an ablation or device implant, I often hear tunes ranging from Fleetwood Mac to U2 to Ed Sheeran. Trust me, it's not for my benefit. The music is for the person on the table, who is understandably anxious and nervous regarding the procedure that is about to happen. Music reorients the brain to the bigger picture of life. The music takes us out of our repetitive thought loops and stories to an emotional release. Depending on the song, that emotional release may be joy, sorrow, anger, or pure energy.

Classical music, in particular, has been shown to have plenty of health benefits including lowering blood pressure and heart rate. For example, H. J. Trappe and colleagues of Ruhr-University Bochum conducted a randomized, controlled study of sixty subjects who were exposed to one of three musical compositions by Mozart, Strauss, or ABBA. There was also a control group of sixty subjects, who rested in silence. Blood pressure, heart rate, and cortisol levels were analyzed. The researchers found a statistically significant reduction in blood pressure, heart rate, and serum cortisol levels, which were greatest in the classical music groups, who listened to Mozart and Strauss. The group who listened to Mozart, in this case it was Symphony No. 40 in G minor, had the greatest effect with these biometrics: a 4.7 point drop in systolic blood pressure, for example. Given the characteristics of the Mozart piece, the scientists suggested that in order for music to reduce blood pressure, it should have no lyrics, have few changes in rhythm or volume, have harmonies that are "not rousing," and that certain parts of the music should be repeated in intervals.

Tool #5: Nutrition

The Greek physician Hippocrates once said, "Let food be thy medicine and medicine be thy food." And it is so true. As I mentioned earlier, excessive caffeine and alcohol consumption is definitely a trigger for AFib. Furthermore, a diet high in carbohydrates and saturated fats can contribute to heart disease and diabetes. I generally recommend the Mediterranean diet to most of my patients, since there is a lot of data showing its health benefits, for not only heart disease, but cancer prevention and other conditions as well. The Mediterranean diet emphasizes eating plant-based foods, such as fruits, vegetables, whole grains, legumes, and nuts.

It also suggests replacing butter with healthy fats such as olive oil, using herbs and spices in place of salt to flavor foods, limiting red meat to no more than a few times a month, and eating fish and poultry at least twice a week, which can be substituted with other proteins such as tofu in patients who are vegetarian or vegan. You may want to consider incorporating some foods high in magnesium and potassium to preserve electrolytes and help reduce premature beats, as long as your kidney function is reasonable, as assessed by your doctor. These foods include kelp, wheat bran, almonds, cashews, millet, walnuts, tofu, rye, soybeans, figs, collard greens, avocado, beans, barley, and garlic. I do believe that there is merit in certain holistic supplements—such as ginger and turmeric—as anti-inflammatory agents. However, there is no concrete scientific data that any one food reduces the chances of atrial fibrillation episodes. Yet, a diet that is geared toward achieving and maintaining an ideal body weight reduces the risk of obesity, which evidently is associated with AFib. So, this gets back to risk-factor modification.

Tool #6: Sleep

Good sleep hygiene is fundamental for our health. Sleep is one of the most restorative processes for our bodies. It is a time for rest, recovery, and rebuilding. Take magnesium before bedtime, avoid smartphones and computers in the evening, read a book or listen to calming music before bedtime, or try one of the many sleep apps on the market. I can't begin to tell you how many times I hear a story from a patient where the AFib event was partially triggered by lack of sleep. Poor sleep is associated with elevated levels of stress hormones, elevated blood pressure, increased irritability and mood lability, and difficulty concentrating. Sleep is one of the biggest parts of developing resilience in life. Challenges seem to loom so much larger when you have poor sleep. After a proper night's rest, challenges become opportunities to learn more.

Tool #7: Social Support System

To keep you accountable for your health, exercise, diet, and sleep, it is important to have accountability partners. These can be friends, family members, colleagues—anyone whom you trust and will be honest with you. Someone who is encouraging and positive is important. It is common when you face an illness to feel alone, so having a social support system in place gives you a group of people you can turn to for moral and physical support. For example, if you are attempting to lose weight and you are trying out a plant-based whole-food plan, doing so with your significant other will increase the likelihood that you both stick with it. Having that friend you meet at 7 a.m. every day to do laps with around the neighborhood keeps you moving in that positive health pattern.

Tool #8: Health Care Team

Your team of doctors, nurses, and allied health professionals represent an important tool in your toolbox. They are a source of information, advice, diagnosis, and treatment. They are partners in your health. It is not a dictatorial system. It is a two-way street. When I first started practicing medicine, I saw my role as an instructor, not a partner. Over the years, I have been humbled time and again by the people who come to my practice and allow me to treat them. And I now realize that people know their own bodies the best, and one of my roles is to mindfully listen first, and give recommendations second.

Completing the Toolbox

So, the idea of having a toolbox in dealing with an illness is really about creating a set of coping strategies when challenges come up. Not mentioned above, but also important, is laughter. In his book *Anatomy of an Illness*, Norman Cousins used laughter to help him on a path to wellness. Cousins would watch episodes of *Candid Camera* and funny movies. He recommends this for all of us whether we are facing a health issue or just living with the stress of everyday modern life. Most of us don't get enough laughter in our lives and should take steps to include this very inexpensive but highly effective method of "healing" ourselves. Some of my favorite comedic movies are *Step Brothers*, *Old School*, the *Pitch Perfect* series, *Trading Places*, and *Zoolander*. You no doubt have your own favorites. I encourage you to have a few laughs each day.

These strategies help build emotional, mental, and physical resilience. Equally important to individual resilience is the concept of connecting with your support network. It is through this approach that you can face anything AFib may throw your way. With all this in mind, it is time to put an action plan to use to get the full range of benefits the toolbox can offer.

Action Plan

1. Write down the 3-Steps to overcoming AFib on a piece of paper and list one short-term and one long-term goal for each.

2. Write down the components of your toolbox. You can include the eight listed in this chapter or incorporate whatever works for you.

3. Write down a list of people you can turn to for support.

CHAPTER 6

Build a Team

"Individual commitment to a group effort—that is what makes a team work, a company work, a society work, a civilization work."

—**Vince Lombardi,** Green Bay Packers
former head coach and football legend

"My heart was pounding and it felt like it was going to jump out of my chest . . . they did the EKG and my heart started to go into AFib again."

—**Billie Jean King,** tennis champion and gender rights crusader

Many different health care providers can be involved in the diagnosis and treatment of atrial fibrillation. The most specialized are cardiac electrophysiologists. These physicians have had specific training and possess significant experience in managing AFib. This ranges from diagnosis to treatment to follow-up. For me, the decision to become a cardiac electrophysiologist really started with my father. As I mentioned, he had heart disease and died suddenly from cardiac arrest. In medical training, I found heart physiology fascinating. In particular, electrophysiology was intellectually stimulating, and EP procedures offered immediate improvement to patients of all ages. Electrical issues of the heart can affect people of any age, from unborn child to centenarian. To find an EP, ask your primary care physician or cardiologist, or to locate an EP directly, go to the Heart Rhythm Society website (hrsonline.org) and click on *find a specialist.* To find an AFib specialist, go to getsmartaboutafib.com and click on *find a doctor.*

What defines a good AFib specialist? Clinical experience, approachability, knowledge base, communication skills, and integrity are some of the most important aspects to consider. While your physician's background training is extremely important, it's how they are now that matters the most. When considering an AFib procedure, you need to find out the number of procedures the physician has performed, the success rates, the complication rates, how endpoints for success are measured, and what the follow-up is like.

In today's health care system, team-based care is the model. The team typically includes a physician, an allied health professional, such as a nurse practitioner or physician assistant, a medical assistant, and the front office staff. The idea is that a patient's visit to the office should have a predictable and comprehensive flow. Allied health professionals should help in the day-to-day communications with patients. Now, this model is best suited for primary care clinics. When you consider advanced subspecialty care, there are some different considerations. Currently, there is a popular movement to form "AFib clinics," which are often run by EP nurse practitioners, and where the coordination of AFib care takes place. These clinics may include a multidisciplinary approach to AFib, with risk-factor modification being a critical part of managing the disease. For this approach, a clinic could partner with sleep specialists, nutritionists, endocrinologists, cardiologists, and neurologists.

That being said, you don't have to wait for an AFib clinic to come your way. You can assemble your team proactively. You have a right to ask your health care providers to communicate with each other if you feel caught in the middle.

Who else should be on your team? Your support network of family and friends and perhaps other patients with atrial fibrillation. Many of my patients find that the discussion boards on websites like stopafib.org are helpful because they can run things by other people who have faced this disease.

Action Plan

1. Go to the Heart Rhythm Society website (hrsonline.org) and find an EP specialist in your area. Use valuation search engines such as Healthgrades (healthgrades.com) and Vitals (vitals.com) to look at reviews on physicians you are considering.

2. Talk to friends, family, and colleagues about who they would recommend as an AFib specialist. Nurses who work with EP specialists are another good source. At your local hospital, ask nurses in the cardiology outpatient units or cath lab. If you know anyone in the medical device industry (Medtronic, Boston Scientific, Abbott, Biosense Webster), ask if they have good recommendations based on working with certain physicians.

3. Make an appointment. Make sure to include your health care team in the decision-making process.

BE IN
CONTROL

CHAPTER 7

Be Watchful

*"There are times where fear is good. It must keep
its watchful place at the heart's controls."*

—**Aeschylus,** ancient Greek writer

*"Atrial fibrillation has been the low man on the totem pole and so
we're just trying to get more visibility about this particular disease
and how dangerous this could be."*

—**Barry Manilow,** singer-songwriter

Monitoring AFib is critical in managing the disease, and I've mentioned throughout this book that AFib is progressive. Each episode of AFib changes the cellular matrix in the electrical system to facilitate having more episodes: AFib begets AFib. For this reason, it is very important to have a way of monitoring the frequency and duration of episodes. Additional quantitative data such as the average heart rate during AFib has merit because chronically elevated rates can weaken the heart muscle—a phenomenon known as a tachycardia cardiomyopathy.

There are many ways to monitor the status of your AFib. A lot of it has to do with what types of symptoms you may or may not have. Some people keep a diary of symptoms: time, date, duration, triggers, and treatments. Others use basic monitors such as blood pressure machines that detect an irregular pulse. There are several devices on the market that can do a single-electrode EKG recording. The most well known and validated is the Kardia device by AliveCor. This device includes a finger sensor and Bluetooth interface with a smartphone. The device will do a real-time recording of the heart's rhythm. The recording will then be classified as normal, undetermined, or atrial fibrillation. The most common reason for undetermined rhythms is either electrical noise from poor electrode contact or frequent premature beats. One can pay for a service whereby a physician will review and interpret the tracings. Alternatively, you can show your AFib specialist the recordings. In clinical studies, the sensitivity of the test is around 90 percent and the specificity is around 80 percent with a good negative predictive value.

Apple has released a software update for the Apple Watch Series 4, which has been cleared by the FDA. This software update allows the wearer to perform a real-time single-lead EKG by placing a finger on a sensor embedded in the side of the watch face. This is useful if someone is having symptoms of palpitations and wants a real-time assessment to see if there may be AFib present. Some criticize the technology, noting that in some of the published data there was a high rate of false positives. Apple submitted a study to the FDA stating that it can detect AFib 99 percent of the time when it can get a reading. That being said, the positive predictive value is only 45 percent. That means the likelihood that an alert is accurate is only 45 percent, meaning in 55 percent of cases an alert was labeled as AFib, but in fact was not.

Apple Watches that are Series 1 and higher have an optical sensor that can detect irregularities in heart rhythm throughout the day without a person needing to actively record anything. In fact, Stanford University has announced a study to examine the ability of the Apple Watch to detect AFib. This study, known as the Apple Heart Study, is a single-arm, pragmatic study that has enrolled 419,093 participants, all of whom have Apple 1 or higher models and an iPhone.

If a sufficient number of irregular pulse events are detected by the watch, the study participant receives a notification and is asked to schedule a visit with a doctor in the study. The participants are then sent EKG rhythm patch monitors to see how many of the people with pulse irregularity notifications by the watch actually have AFib episodes on the patch. Secondary objectives of the study are: (1) to examine the relationship between watch notifications and simultaneous patch recordings, and (2) to assess the rate of initial contact with a health care provider within three months after watch notification. Participants interface with study physicians via a telemedicine interface.

As described in Chapter 2, there are several different types of medical rhythm monitors: Holter, event recorder, mobile telemetry, and patch monitors. The patch monitor is a decent option to peri-odically check for any silent episodes of AFib a person may not feel yet, but which may still cause progression of the disease.

Implantable loop monitors are the most advanced form of rhythm monitoring. These have the advantage of continuous remote monitoring with a battery life of three years, and the abil-ity to detect silent AFib. Signals are sent to physicians via a home monitoring box interfacing with cell phone towers. If we use the analogy mentioned before that AFib is like electrical cancer, then the implantable loop monitor can be thought of as a way to moni-tor this cancer. This is similar to a colonoscopy for colon cancer or mammogram for breast cancer.

The last way of monitoring atrial fibrillation is through pace-makers and defibrillators, if patients have those implanted for other reasons. These devices have sophisticated algorithms to detect atrial fibrillation, including time of day, duration, and amount, which is called percent burden.

Action Plan

1. Start a diary of AFib episodes including time of day, duration, frequency, triggers, and treatment. Identify the patterns.

2. Check out wearable and smartphone-enabled rhythm monitors. Go to the Apple store to have a demonstration of Apple Watch Series 4 EKG. Go to alivecor.com to try out the Kardia device. Because of their health application, these devices may qualify as out-of-pocket health care expenses for a health saving plan or itemized tax deduction. Please consult with an expert in these areas to know for sure. Learn more about implantable loop monitors by visiting medtronic.com.

CHAPTER 8

Be Updated

*"Rhythm is something you either have or don't have,
but when you have it, you have it all over."*

—Elvis Presley, musician and actor

*"Persistent atrial fibrillation . . . which the doctors told me could
have been the end of my career. I had four weeks of complete rest and
treatment . . . I can enjoy cycling like never before."*

—Haimar Zubeldia, professional road racing cyclist champion

I t is imperative to stay abreast of the latest developments in
atrial fibrillation diagnosis and treatment. Often, your physician may not be able to keep up with everything. Thus, it is
incumbent upon you to take charge of your condition and stay
up-to-date. This will help to facilitate a dialogue with your health

care provider. Several reputable websites are in place to keep you informed of the latest in understanding AFib and technological developments, as well as cutting-edge research (see below). Some include forums for people to discuss topics and stories (remember, one must be careful in generalizing one person's experience to others). I have found four websites, in particular, to be useful for patients in staying up-to-date on their AFib: StopAfib.org, getsmartaboutafib.com, hrsonline.org (Heart Rhythm Society), and heart.org (American Heart Association).

StopAfib.org

This organization was founded in 2007 by Mellanie True Hills, a corporate executive, who developed atrial fibrillation and eventually underwent a "mini-maze" surgical AFib ablation procedure. When she finally knew what life was like living without atrial fibrillation, she wanted to create something that could help others afflicted with this disease. StopAfib.org is a nonprofit organization that educates and supports atrial fibrillation patients and their family members. The website is packed with original and curated AFib content describing the condition, explaining why it is a problem, and offering several additional resources for further study. The "Can AFib Be Cured?" section offers descriptions of different treatment options. The "Patient Stories" section is where real people share their experiences with AFib.

The site also features an AFib specialist finder, as well as discussion forums where patients can share experiences and ask questions. The StopAfib organization has partnered with several international professional medical organizations and patient organizations to raise awareness of AFib and advocate for patients worldwide. An annual atrial fibrillation patient conference is hosted that brings together leading world experts on AFib. StopAfib.org has collaborated with the Alliance for Aging Research on their Year Without a Stroke campaign, an effort to share stories of people who have experienced, and seen firsthand, how serious AFib-related strokes can be. One of StopAfib's goals is to raise awareness of AFib, so those who have it, but don't realize it, get diagnosed and treated before they have a stroke. You can sign up for email alerts to keep you up-to-date on the latest news with AFib. StopAfib.org and the American Heart Association are co-collaborators on MyAFibExperience.org, which also has AFib content and a discussion forum.

Getsmartaboutafib.com

This website was created by Biosense Webster, Inc., in a joint effort with Stopafib.org, to educate Americans about atrial fibrillation and the treatment options available. Biosense Webster is a leading company in the field of arrhythmia treatment, particularly catheter mapping and ablation technology. The site is interactive, with several video clips and tutorials. Although the site is created by industry, it does project a relatively unbiased view of the disease and treatment options. The "Find a Doctor" section allows you to locate an AFib specialist closest to you by zip code. The site also has helpful materials, such as a list of good questions to ask at the clinic visit.

Heart Rhythm Society

Hrsonline.org is the official website of the Heart Rhythm Society, the international professional organization for heart rhythm specialists, including cardiac electrophysiology physicians, allied health professionals, and researchers. It is a nonprofit organization that promotes education and advocacy for cardiac arrhythmia professionals and patients. The "Patient Resources" section of the website has medical information for patients including normal heart function, risk factors and prevention, heart diseases and disorders, substances and heart rhythm disorders, symptoms and diagnosis, treatment, and patient information sheets. I believe the information on substances and heart rhythm disorders is critical to find out if something you are eating or drinking could contribute to AFib episodes. There is also a "Find a Specialist" search engine for locating an AFib specialist, as well as a helpful glossary of terms section listed in the "Patient Toolkit."

American Heart Association

The American Heart Association (www.heart.org/en/health-topics/atrial-fibrillation) has several online resources for patients with AFib. The site is sectioned into these topics: (1) What is atrial fibrillation, (2) Why atrial fibrillation matters, (3) What are the symptoms of atrial fibrillation, and (4) Treatment and prevention of atrial fibrillation. There is also a "Starting Question" you can submit to get you on the path of education. It presents the question: "What is the biggest challenge you or a loved one faces following an atrial fibrillation diagnosis?" The options for responses include the following: (1) No one understands what I am going through, (2) I need help modifying my lifestyle to better manage AFib, (3) I'm worried about my increased risk for stroke, and (4) I'm not sure what my treatment options are. Once you select one of the responses, the site will take you through a series of pages specifically targeted to answer the question. This is very helpful when it comes to navigating websites that have a lot of information, which can be overwhelming to say the least.

Action Plan

1. Begin investigating some patient-friendly websites to get updated information about atrial fibrillation.

2. Sign up to receive alerts about AFib ranging from diagnostic technologies to new treatment options. Stopafib.org is a good option for this.

3. Make it a habit to check websites every three months regarding updates.

CHAPTER 9

Be the Master

"It is not in the stars to hold our destiny but in ourselves."
—**William Shakespeare,** English poet and playwright

This chapter is about summing it all up. Be the master of your health. Be informed, be proactive, be confident, be humble, be vulnerable, and be with others. The key with atrial fibrillation is early detection and early intervention. It is like electrical cancer. If detected and treated early, the long-term maintenance of sinus rhythm is high and the recurrence rate will be lower compared to AFib that has progressed. However, even patients with persistent atrial fibrillation and long-standing persistent atrial fibrillation have treatment options.

Remember, when it comes to overcoming anything, we are

not necessarily talking about a cure. We are talking about facing a challenge head-on and using it as an opportunity for growth. Perhaps the challenge can even be used as an opportunity to help others in their battle with this electrical chaos.

To summarize, cardiac arrhythmias are due to three mechanisms: reentry, triggered activity, and automaticity. There are three types of atrial fibrillation: paroxysmal (comes and goes, self-terminates), persistent (continuous, less than one year, requires intervention such as cardioversion), long-standing persistent (over one year), and permanent (treatment decision between doctor and patient that the risk of intervention is greater than the risk of the condition). Risk factors for atrial fibrillation include age over sixty-five, high blood pressure, diabetes, obesity, and sleep apnea. Emerging risk factors may also include certain genetic mutations (cardiac sodium channel) and high-endurance athleticism with associated bradycardia (low heart rate). Triggers for atrial fibrillation include electrolyte deficiency (especially magnesium and potassium), dehydration, alcohol, caffeine, poor sleep, and stress. Often a "perfect storm" of these results in a specific episode.

Diagnosis of atrial fibrillation can be done with a variety of rhythm-recording devices: electrocardiogram (EKG), Holter monitor (forty-eight hours), telemetry monitor (four weeks), Zio patch monitor (two weeks), implantable loop monitor (three years, continuous data collection), wearable monitors (Apple Watch Series 4 EKG feature), and smartphone-enabled (Kardia by AliveCor). Wearable monitors and smartphone devices are limited in that they are only helpful if a patient is in AFib at the time of the recording.

Once a diagnosis is confirmed, workup includes ruling out structural heart disease with echocardiography and stress testing. After this, trigger elimination and risk factor modification are implemented to see if episodes decrease. If the episodes continue, therapeutic options include drug therapy, cardioversion, pacing, and ablation. Drugs include rate control agents (beta-blockers, calcium channel blockers) and antiarrhythmic drugs (propafenone, flecainide, amiodarone, dofetilide, sotalol, dronedarone, and disopyramide). Cardioversion is used to restore the rhythm but does not prevent future episodes of atrial fibrillation.

Newer pacemakers have the ability to terminate atrial fibrillation episodes with antitachycardia pacing and suppress premature atrial contractions from triggering AFib by overdrive pacing. Leadless pacemakers are now available for select patients. Atrial fibrillation ablation remains the most effective modality to maintain sinus rhythm. Radiofrequency and cryo energy are the two most commonly used. Sometimes a combination of approaches is undertaken, especially in long-standing persistent atrial fibrillation. Left atrial enlargement and left atrial scarring are important predictors of arrhythmia recurrence. Risk-factor modification reduces the recurrence rate of atrial fibrillation after ablation. New hybrid ablation procedures such as Convergent Procedure appear to offer benefit in patients with refractory atrial fibrillation.

In patients where the goal is normal sinus rhythm, I will restate a concept I mentioned earlier. The bottom line with AFib is that it does not matter how to get to maintaining sinus rhythm (meds, ablation, device, combination); the treatment is being in sinus rhythm. Again, just as AFib begets AFib, sinus rhythm begets sinus rhythm. The heart is a muscle, and being in AFib creates a muscle memory that makes the heart want to stay in AFib. We just need to change the default muscle memory to that of sinus rhythm. And the longer the heart remains in sinus, the lower the chances of recurrent AFib. As I've said, every day of sinus rhythm is a good day and one to celebrate—don't look too far into the future.

The most important thing about atrial fibrillation is knowing that no two people with atrial fibrillation have the same disease, many treatment options are available, and treatment must be tailored to the patient.

Action Plan

1. Repeat to yourself: AFib begets AFib.

2. Repeat to yourself: sinus rhythm begets sinus rhythm.

3. Repeat to yourself: early detection and early intervention are crucial.

Conclusion

One of the greatest challenges with AFib is how it varies individual to individual. This is the case with all types of AFib. People vary in their risk factors, triggers, associated diseases, ages, and individual cardiac anatomy and electrophysiology. It is important to keep this in mind when comparing experiences with others with AFib. Treating AFib is really about treating the big picture: all parts of the mind and body working together. The brain-heart connection is increasingly being recognized as critical in arrhythmia medicine.

Take-Home Points

1. There is significant misinformation about AFib. Be discerning of what you read and hear.

2. AFib can affect anyone. It is a systemic disease ranging from genetics to risk factors to age-related scarring.

3. AFib is an individual disease that varies from individual to individual. It requires a tailored approach to each person.

4. There are multiple treatment options for AFib. The key is to have realistic expectations of what and what cannot be done in today's world. That means becoming educated. More and more people have been able to get into sinus rhythm with the advancements in understanding of the disease and technology. Treatments may differ depending on the type of AFib, age, and accompanying comorbidities. Treatments may be individual therapies such as ablation, drugs, or devices, or a combination of these. The final common pathway for treatment is maintaining normal sinus rhythm. That creates the new muscle memory required to keep the disease at bay.

5. AFib is electrical cancer. Early detection and intervention are critical. There are various technologies available and emerging to help diagnose AFib and monitor the disease. Treatments become less effective as the disease progresses.

6. For the best possible outcome, all risk factors and triggers for AFib must be optimized. AFib is often part of a larger metabolic dysregulation. Any treatment is less effective when the body is out of balance.

7. The brain-heart connection via the autonomic nervous system is integral in AFib. The whole body needs to be balanced to have the best outcome with AFib.

8. Medical therapy for AFib has not had any significant advancements in decades. The biggest limitation with drugs is that they are not specific for the atria but can affect the ventricles and other organs as well.

9. Ablation today is far more successful and has less risk than ever before. Education, risk-factor and trigger modification, and patient selection is critical.

10. The treatment of AFib is multidisciplinary. There is an emerging movement to have AFib "clinics" where education and risk-factor modification take place (sleep apnea screening and treatment, weight loss programs, etc.).

11. Overcoming AFib may mean something different to each person, whether it be elimination of events, a reduction in events and improved quality of life, or staying in AFib and having protection against stroke and congestive heart failure.

12. Widespread education of the public, patients, health care professionals, health care systems, and insurance companies is critical. Ignorance breeds ignorance. Up-to-date education breeds informed decisions about health.

Case Studies

"The moment you breathe your first breath, you won."

—J. R. Rim, author

Sometimes, it is helpful to understand a disease and options when hearing stories from other people. Let's hear some stories about people like you and me, who have been affected by AFib—and their stories in overcoming it. These stories represent real people with AFib, whom I have had the privilege of partnering with to improve their lives. To protect patient privacy, their names have been changed and there is no identifying information in accordance with HIPAA (the Health Insurance Portability and Accounting Act).

Two Birds with One Stone

Chris is an eighteen-year-old, healthy college student, though with a family history of cardiac arrhythmias. One day, he experienced sudden unbearable heart racing and dizziness. It terrified him and his family. He went to the emergency room after calling 911 and was found to be in AFib. It wasn't clear what triggered it. He was healthy, with no individual history of heart disease. He had skipping heartbeats on and off for a few years and was told it was "benign." His father had a history of AFib that started at age forty.

Chris's caffeine and alcohol intake were not significant. His heart was structurally normal on echo and stress testing. A rhythm monitor detected two abnormal rhythms—supraventricular tachycardia (SVT) and atrial fibrillation. (SVT episodes can trigger atrial fibrillation.) He tried metoprolol—a beta-blocker medication—but felt extremely fatigued and had insomnia with it. He tried flecainide and had severe headaches. Chris's quality of life was terrible. He was afraid to hang out with his friends for fear of going out of rhythm and having to go to the emergency room.

He couldn't travel with his family because he never knew when his heart was going to "act up," as he called it. I discussed the idea of catheter ablation with Chris early on but didn't want to push it too hard because I could sense he was overwhelmed. Mutual trust is the cornerstone of the doctor-patient relationship. I have often found that some people need to hit a certain threshold of events to help them move to the next step in treatment.

One day, Chris was taking his final exams and could feel himself going into SVT. He tried the maneuvers he was taught to terminate the event (holding his breath, coughing, bearing down) but they were unsuccessful. He felt the "switch" in rhythm from a regular rapid pulse to something completely chaotic in his chest. His school called 911 and he was subsequently cardioverted in the ER for atrial fibrillation. This was it for Chris. He needed to do something so that he was not consumed with this disease.

He underwent a successful ablation procedure—in fact, the cause of his AFib was SVT due to what is called a concealed accessory pathway. This is an extra connection of electrical tissue that can cause a reentrant arrhythmia called orthodromic reciprocating tachycardia. During the procedure, the SVT repetitively transitioned to AFib, so it was clear that SVT was the driving rhythm abnormality.

After the pathway was successfully ablated, no atrial fibrillation could be induced. This was life-changing for Chris. He could feel his heart was immediately "calm" after the procedure. He used to get skipping heartbeats all the time. Now, he was no longer aware of his heartbeat, and that was such a nice feeling to have. Chris went on to pursue a career in medicine and eventually became a physician assistant with a focus in cardiology. He feels tremendous empathy for his patients because he knows firsthand what it is like to feel a broken heart, and have it healed again.

Out of the Fog, Into the Light

Kelsey is a forty-year-old, successful real estate agent without any history of heart disease. However, one day she experienced profound and unexplainable fatigue. Subsequently, she would have these "waves" of fatigue—some days she would feel great and other days terrible. Depression got the better of her, and she withdrew from life. She felt her breath fade. She was otherwise healthy, so she only saw a physician on an as-needed basis, such as when she had bronchitis. Finally, her husband pleaded with her to see a doctor.

The doctor listened to her heart and heard a very irregular rhythm. The EKG showed atrial fibrillation. Kelsey said, "I don't even feel my heart beating funny—could this be causing my depression?" She thought some of her fatigue and mood was related to the heavy stress she was under at her job. She subsequently had a Zio patch monitor that correlated the days she felt poorly to the days she was in AFib. There were times she was in AFib for up to four days. Because she was so young, she was not interested in trying out medication that she would have to take long term. She wanted a more definitive strategy. Kelsey underwent a cryoballoon pulmonary vein isolation ablation. During the procedure, when the fourth pulmonary vein was electrically isolated, her AFib immediately converted to a normal sinus rhythm.

She has not had a single episode of AFib since then. Her mood lifted and she felt like she came out of a "fog." Before her bouts of fatigue, Kelsey was running four to five miles several days a week. When she developed AFib, that stopped. Now, she is able to run up to seven miles and is scheduled to do her first half marathon in a few months. Kelsey purchased a Kardia device to track her rhythm every day. She joined stopafib.org and interacts with other members of the community, offering words of encouragement to people who are where Kelsey has been before: defeated, dejected, ready to give up. Kelsey says, "It may not be the same as my case, but it is definitely worth getting evaluated by a specialist for your AFib."

Go after the Second-in-Command

Tom is a sixty-year-old physician with a history of high blood pressure. He is also an avid runner. Tom has helped many people improve their health. Yet one day, he found himself on the other side, as a patient being rushed to the emergency room. His breathing became shallow during the ambulance ride, and his head was spinning with thoughts of what was going to happen. Earlier in the day, he was seeing patients in the office when he suddenly felt very dizzy. In the ER he was found to be in AFib. They gave him intravenous diltiazem, which converted him to a normal rhythm. There was no obvious trigger to the AFib.

He kept having recurrent episodes, so he was prescribed metoprolol and it worked well for several years. Since Tom knew AFib was a progressive disease and there was such a thing called silent AFib, he wanted to have a way to track the episodes in terms of duration and frequency. He had an implantable loop monitor placed. The device showed he was having significantly more episodes of AFib than he thought. He subsequently started having more symptomatic episodes despite the metoprolol. Concerned about the side effects of antiarrhythmic medication and possible proarrhythmia, he underwent a pulmonary vein isolation procedure with non-contact force-sensing radiofrequency technology (the contact force-sensing was not available yet). He did well for about one year, then had recurrence. He underwent a second ablation. Here, some of the AFib was found to be due to pulmonary vein reconnection.

However, Tom had a new trigger not seen on the first ablation: the superior vena cava vein. This represented what is called an extra pulmonary vein trigger. Often these triggers are not seen at the first ablation because the pulmonary veins overshadow them. Once the pulmonary veins were electrically isolated and the SVC was also isolated, Tom's AFib diminished significantly. While his AFib did not completely resolve, his episodes were far less frequent and milder, thereby improving his quality of life.

Fear Is Just a Four-Letter Word

Pat is an eighty-nine-year-old retired schoolteacher who volunteers at a nearby hospital. She has a history of diabetes, sleep apnea, and coronary artery bypass surgery. She experienced chronic general malaise that she attributed to getting older. It was almost as if she couldn't take a deep breath. Like something was restricting her. It terrified her and kept her in a constant state of worry. She wore a telemetry monitor, which demonstrated episodes of rapid atrial fibrillation and atrial flutter that were causing these symptoms.

This was occurring despite her being on both metoprolol and diltiazem. What was interesting was that she did not experience a fast or irregular heartbeat. When we met in the office after the monitor results, we first examined her triggers and risk factors and optimized those. This included reducing caffeine intake, being more aggressive about blood pressure management, and achieving some weight loss. However, she continued to have very symptomatic episodes, so we moved to the next step. Pat wanted to try an antiarrhythmic drug first. Because of her coronary artery disease history and already being on a beta-blocker, our choices were limited to dofetilide, amiodarone, and dronedarone. Dronedarone is known to cause significant gastrointestinal distress, and Pat has a history of irritable bowel syndrome.

She preferred to avoid amiodarone at all costs based on what she knew about its side effects. She elected for dofetilide. Dofetilide did control her AFib well for about six months, but then she started having breakthrough episodes. Pat ultimately underwent two AFib ablations. Though she remains on a low dose of dofetilide, she is completely free of AFib and feels like she has a new lease on life. With the last ablation, she had an implantable monitor placed, so now she doesn't have to worry about whether she is in AFib because she knows our office is monitoring it. She previously would not want to travel with her husband for fear of going into AFib. Now she doesn't even think about it.

Size Is Only a Number

Jack is a pleasant, sixty-five-year-old man whom I met about three years ago. He is a part of a group of friends who all have AFib. They were friends for other reasons, of course, but they coincidentally found this common denominator in their health. Jack married his childhood sweetheart and they have been together for forty lovely years. He and his wife love to travel and they enjoy learning about and trying different wines. Jack began developing episodes of shortness of breath, and despite having several diagnostic tests, the cause could not be determined.

One day he showed up at his primary care physician's office in rapid AFib. At that point it was unclear how long it had been going on. His echo showed a severely enlarged left atrium, which suggested the AFib had already caused a fair amount of scarring and damage. So, Jack was diagnosed with persistent AFib of unknown duration. I met with him and his wife and we talked about treatment options at length. I explained that with a very large left atrium, the recurrence rate of AFib is high with any intervention.

We talked about how it was more of a process in knocking down this opponent. Jack wanted to try a cardioversion first just to see if he felt any better in sinus rhythm, even if it lasted for a day. He underwent a successful cardioversion and for four days he felt amazing; then the AFib recurred. Jack felt that trying different medications with different side effects was not the direction he wanted to go in life. He knew ablation had its limitations with the amount of atrial enlargement he had, but he decided to take a leap of faith. His first ablation was coupled with the use of dofetilide for six months after. He did well in sinus rhythm for about a year and then had a recurrence. Initially, he was able to limit AFib episodes when he stopped drinking the wine he and his wife loved so much. Ultimately, the AFib broke through again.

He underwent a second ablation, and an implantable monitor was placed to track the rhythm. The monitor revealed multiple pauses in the heartbeat that would occur during times AFib converted to sinus rhythm. These are known as post-conversion pauses, and they typically happen when the sinus node function is abnormal. He would get extremely lightheaded during these events. Ultimately, a pacemaker was implanted. This pacemaker had a special algorithm for suppressing AFib by detecting premature atrial beats and suppressing them with atrial pacing. Furthermore, it also had an algorithm to terminate episodes of atrial flutter by pacing faster than the atrial flutter arrhythmia, essentially overriding the circuit. With the combination of ablation, medication, and pacing, Jack is now someone with severe left atrial enlargement who is living in sinus rhythm.

He was told by several people that his chances of getting here were slim to none. But Jack's spirit was strong, and he didn't give up the fight. And as a result of Jack giving up wine, he lost fifteen pounds and has more energy now than he has had in twenty years.

The Takeaway

All of the above stories illustrate how AFib is a condition, whose treatment needs to be individualized to a person's specific triggers, AFib risk factors, and associated arrhythmias. In some patients, trigger modification is enough. In others, managing risk factors such as high blood pressure and sleep apnea can make the difference. For some, medication is the way to go. For others, ablation. In more advanced cases, ablation may be an option via a hybrid endocardial-surgical approach. Yet, in some cases, a pacemaker plus meds works. Lastly, in some patients a pacemaker, meds, and pulmonary vein ablation is the magic formula, so to speak.

Glossary

Antitachycardia pacing (ATP)—a feature on implantable devices, which can terminate arrhythmias by causing a block of electrical impulses in a reentrant circuit by overdriving them.

Arrhythmia—abnormal heart rhythm, usually classified as tachycardia (fast) or bradycardia (slow). Also includes premature beats and atrial fibrillation.

Atrial fibrillation (AFib)—a condition whereby the top chambers of the heart quiver in a rapid uncoordinated fashion up to 600 beats per minute. This can lead to stagnation of blood and the formation of a clot, which can cause a stroke among other sequelae. It is the most common cardiac arrhythmia worldwide.

AV node—a group of cells in the center of the electrical system. They act as a "tollbooth" controlling impulses from going too fast from top to bottom of the heart.

Cardiac electrophysiologist—a cardiologist with specialized training and experience in diagnosing and treating cardiac arrhythmias—most notably atrial fibrillation.

Congestive heart failure (CHF)—a syndrome that includes symptoms such as shortness of breath and volume retention related to a weakened heart muscle (systolic CHF) or stiff heart muscle (diastolic CHF).

Electrophysiology study (EPS)—a procedure in which catheters are placed in the electrical system of the heart to diagnose and treat heart rhythm disorders.

Heart attack—the acute formation of a blood clot in one or more of the three coronary arteries resulting in cell and tissue death of a certain part of the heart muscle.

Long-standing persistent atrial fibrillation—persistent AFib lasting more than one year.

Normal sinus rhythm—the definition of a normal electrical rhythm in the heart. The heartbeat originates in a group of cells called the sinus node.

Pacemaker—a medical device used primarily to treat a slow heart rate with associated symptoms.

Paroxysmal atrial fibrillation—a type of AFib defined as self-terminating without the need for a medical intervention. Typically, episodes are less than forty-eight hours.

Permanent atrial fibrillation—a decision made by doctor and patient to stay in AFib and focus on heart rate control because the risk of any intervention to maintain normal sinus rhythm is felt to be greater than the likelihood and benefit of normal sinus rhythm.

Persistent atrial fibrillation—a type of AFib defined as continuous for longer than one week, which requires a medical intervention, like cardioversion, to terminate.

Premature atrial contraction (PAC)—an extra heartbeat originating from the top chambers of the heart. Often triggered by excessive caffeine, alcohol, dehydration, or stress.

Pulmonary veins—four vessels that bring back oxygenated blood from the lungs to the left atrium. They contain muscular sleeves that connect to the left atrium proper. These sleeves contain electrical cells that feature all three mechanisms of arrhythmias—automaticity, triggered activity, and reentry.

Reentry—a mechanism of cardiac arrhythmias by which a vicious loop of electrical impulse movement is created. Examples include supraventricular tachycardia and atrial flutter.

Sinus node—a group of cells at the top part of the right atrium, which sets the heartbeat. These cells are influenced by states of adrenaline.

Bibliography

American Heart Association. "Kenley Jansen Pitches an Important Message to Everyone." https://www.heart.org/en/health-topics/ atrial-fibrillation/afib-resources-for-patients--professionals/ kenley-jansen-pitches-an-important-message-to-everyone.

Berman, M. G., et al. "The Cognitive Benefits of Interacting with Nature." *Psychological Science* (2008) 19 (12): 1207–1212.

Cousins, Norman. *Anatomy of an Illness as Perceived by the Patient: Reflections on Healing.* New York: W. W. Norton, 1979.

Cycling News. "Zubeldia Discloses Cardiac Problems in Early 2012." Future PLC. July 22, 2012. https://www.cyclingnews.com/news/ zubeldia-discloses-cardiac-problems-in-early-2012.

Daily Headbänger. "KISS' Gene Simmons Brings Attention to Atrial Fibrillation during Episode of 'The Doctors.'" DotcomCowgirl Media. March 10, 2016. https://dailyheadbanger.com/kiss-gene-simmons-brings-attention-to-atrial-fibrillation-during-episode-of-the-doctors.

Fell, James C. *Los Angeles Times.* "Comic Kevin Nealon Is Still 'Pumped Up' About Fitness." July 3, 2015. https://www.latimes.com/health/la-he-kevin-nealon-interview-20150704-story.html.

Desai, A. D., et al. "The Role of Intravenous Amiodarone in the Management of Cardiac Arrhythmias." *Annals of Internal Medicine* (August 15, 1997) 127 (4): 294–303.

Dewland, T. A., et al. "Atrial Ectopy as a Predictor of Incident Atrial Fibrillation: A Cohort Study." *Annals of Internal Medicine* (2013) 159; 11: 721–728.

Everyday Health. "How Howie Mandel Deals with Atrial Fibrillation." November 14, 2017. https://www.everydayhealth.com/heart-health/ atrial-fibrillation/how-howie-mandel-deals-with-atrial-fibrillation.

Gawande, Atul. *The Checklist Manifesto: How to Get Things Right.* New York: Henry Holt, 2009.

Jacobs, T. L., et al. "Intensive Meditation Training, Immune Cell Telomerase Activity, and Psychological Mediators." *Psychoneuroendocrinology* (2011) 36; 5: 664–681.

Kannell, W. B. "Epidemiology of Atrial Fibrillation: Risk Factors and Hazards." 1st Virtual Congress of Cardiology, 2000.

Kuck, K. H., et al. "Cryoballoon or Radiofrequency Ablation for Paroxysmal Atrial Fibrillation." *New England Journal of Medicine* (2016) 374: 2235–2245.

Lombardi, F., et al. "Acupuncture for Paroxysmal and Persistent Atrial Fibrillation: An Effective Non-pharmacological Tool?" *World Journal of Cardiology* (2012): 60–65.

Lakkireddy, D., et al. "Effect of Yoga on Arrhythmia Burden, Anxiety, Depression, and Quality of Life in Paroxysmal Atrial Fibrillation." *Journal of the American College of Cardiology* (2013) 61; 11: 1177–1182.

McCallum, Jack. Sports Illustrated Vault. "Secrets of the Heart: Larry Bird Reveals That He Has Long Suffered from a Cardiac Condition." TI Gotham Inc. September 6, 1999. https://www.si.com/vault/1999/09/06/8110354/ secrets-of-the-heart-larry-bird-reveals-that-he-has-long-suffered-from-a- cardiac-condition.

Medical Device Network. "J&J to Study Apple Watch in Heart Health Research Project." Verdict Media Limited. January 18, 2019. https://www. medicaldevice-network.com/news/jj-apple-watch-heart-health-study.

Mindful. "Jon Kabat Zinn: Defining Mindfulness." Foundation for a Mindful Society. January 11, 2017. https://www.mindful.org/ jon-kabat-zinn-defining-mindfulness.

Miyasaka, Y., et al. "Secular Trends in Incidence of Atrial Fibrillation in Olmsted County, Minnesota, 1980 to 2000, and Implications on the Projections for Future Prevalence." *Circulation* (July 11, 2006) 114; 2: 119–125.

Novoa, R., et al. "Clinical Hypnosis for Reduction of Atrial Fibrillation after Coronary Artery Bypass Graft Surgery." *Cleveland Clinic Journal of Medicine* (2008) 75 Suppl. 2: S44–47.

Oxford English Dictionary. 2nd Edition. 20 vols. Oxford: Oxford University Press, 1989. Continually updated at https://www.lexico.com/en/definition/overcome.

Rush, Nathan. Athlon Sports. "Tennis Legend Billie Jean King Talks Heart Health and More." Athlon Media Group. February 2, 2016. https://athlonsports.com/life/billie-jean-king-talks-heart-health-and-tennis.

Stanford Medicine. "Stanford, Apple Describe Heart Study with Over 400,000 Participants." November 1, 2018. https://med.stanford.edu/news/all-news/2018/11/stanford-apple-describe-heart-study-with-over-400000-participants.

Sung, R. J., and Lauer, M. R. *Fundamental Approaches to the Management of Cardiac Arrhythmias*. Dordrecht, The Netherlands: Kluwer Academic Publishers, 2000.

Trappe, H. J., et al. "The Cardiovascular Effect of Music Genres: A Randomized Controlled Study on the Effect of Compositions by W. A. Mozart, J. Strauss, and ABBA." *Deutsches Ärzteblatt International* (May 2016) 113 (20): 347–352.

Turakhia, M.P., et al. "Rationale and Design of a Large-Scale, App-Based Study to Identify Cardiac Arrhythmias Using a Smartwatch: The Apple Heart Study." *American Heart Journal* (January 2019) 207: 66–75.

Walker, Matt. "Sleep Is Your Superpower." Filmed April 2019 at a TED conference. https://www.ted.com/talks/matt_walker_sleep_is_your_superpower.

Watts, Alan. *Still the Mind—An Introduction to Meditation*. Novato, California: New World Library, 2000.

Williams, J., et al. "The Effectiveness of a Mobile ECG Device in Identifying AF: Sensitivity, Specificity, and Predictive Value." *British Journal of Cardiology* (2015) 22: 70–72.

Wolf, P. A., et al. "Atrial Fibrillation as an Independent Risk Factor for Stroke: The Framingham Heart Study." *Stroke* (August 1991) 22 (8): 983–988.

Wyse, D. G., et al. "A Comparison of Rate Control and Rhythm Control in Patients with Atrial Fibrillation." *New England Journal of Medicine* (2002) 347: 1825–1833.

Index

An italicized *f* or *t* following a page number refers to a figure or a table respectively.

A

Abbott, 128
ablation. *See* cardiac ablation
accommodation phenomenon, 61
Action Plans, 9, 117, 142, 155, 159–60, 167, 173, 178
acupuncture, 147
adenosine, 101
adrenaline
  abnormal automaticity and, 24–25
  beta-blockers and, 35, 110, 118
  calcium channel blockers and, 112
  dehydration and, 46
  effects on body, 138
  exercise and, 47, 147
  fight-or-flight response, 138
  mindfulness and, 140
  paroxysmal atrial fibrillation and, 65
  SA node and, 18
  sleep apnea and, 37
  sleep hygiene and, 47
  stress and, 48, 142
adrenergic atrial fibrillation, 49
Aeschylus, 163
AFFIRM clinical trial, 87
AFib. *See* atrial fibrillation; heart-rhythm monitoring
aging
  prevalence of AFib by decade of age, 33*f*
  as risk factor, 32, 34
alcohol

reducing, 35, 43
  as trigger, 43–44
AliveCor, 77, 164
Alliance for Aging, 171
Alzheimer's disease, 109, 115
amiodarone (Pacerone), 89*t*, 90–91, 120–22, 189
amlodipine, 35
Anatomy of an Illness (Cousins), 154
Ancient Minerals, 45
ANS (autonomic nervous system), 18, 48, 138, 140, 144, 147, 181
antiarrhythmic drugs, 29, 119–21, 177, 187, 189. *See also names of specific drugs*
  blood pressure drugs, 35
  challenges of, 88
  choosing for treatment, 121–22
  in combination with other treatments, 30
  compared to other treatments, 122
  effects on ion channel receptors, 23
  overview of, 88, 89*t*, 90–91
  potassium channel blockers (class III agents), 89*t*, 90–91, 119–22
  for reentrant arrhythmias, 24
  side effects of, 121
  sodium channel blockers (class Ia/Ic agents), 89*t*, 90, 119–21
  success rate, 90
  for triggered activity arrhythmias, 24

anticoagulants (blood thinners), 73–74, 98, 113, 115, 132
antitachycardia pacing (ATP), 94, 128, 177, 193
aorta, 17*f*
aortic valve, 17*f*
apixaban (Eliquis), 115
Apple Heart Study, 165
Apple Watch, 26, 77, 78*f*, 79, 164–65
arrhythmias, xvi. *See also* antiarrhythmic drugs; *names of specific arrhythmias*
causes of, 23–25, 25*f*, 176
defined, 193
types of, 23
asymptomatic episodes (silent AFib), 60, 66, 69, 72, 75, 166, 187
atenolol (Tenormin), 35, 111*t*, 112, 118
atherosclerosis (coronary artery disease [CAD]), 32, 39–40, 90–91, 119–20, 124, 189
ATP (antitachycardia pacing), 94, 128, 177, 193
atrial fibrillation (AFib), 85. *See also* heart-rhythm monitoring
"AFib begets AFib," 30, 39, 51, 163, 177
analogies
arthritis of the electrical system., 32, 124
broken wires, 27, 29–30
electrical cancer, 8–9, 30, 85, 166, 175, 180
merry-go-round, 24, 28*f*
runner on racetrack, 24, 28*f*, 94
causes of
abnormal cells, 29–30
loss of P wave, 18
nature and nurture, 16, 18, 32
consequences of, xvi, 31
dealing with diagnosis, 137–42
brain-heart connection, 144–45
comparing experiences, 139
deep breathing, 139–40
fight-or-flight response, 138
meditation, 140–41
mindfulness, 140–41
not identifying with AFib, 142
saying it will be okay, 138–39

stress management, 142
toolbox concept, 145–54
defined, 193
diagnosis of, 59–60, 176
asymptomatic episodes, 60
case study, 63–64
echocardiography, 62
electrocardiography, 60–62, 66
heart-rhythm monitoring, 65–66
magnetic resonance imaging, 62–63
pacemakers, 60
panic attacks *vs.*, 60, 65
paroxysmal AFib, 59–60, 65
persistent AFib, 60–62
first event, 8–9
health care team, 157–59
individualized nature of disease and treatment, 7–9, 84, 130, 139, 178–80, 191
keeping up-to-date, 169–73
mass education of health care professionals, 86, 181
overcoming
defined, xv
defining success in overcoming AFib, xv–xvi, 83–85, 175–76, 181
differences in from person to person, 139
prevalence of, 33*f*
projected number of patients with, 33*f*, 34
questions to ask specialist, 81–82
risk factors for, 32–43, 43*f*, 176, 180–81
aging, 32, 33*f*, 34
athleticism, 41–42
congestive heart failure, 40
coronary artery disease, 39–40
diabetes, 39
genetics, 32
high blood pressure, 35–36
obesity, 34–35
premature atrial contractions (PACs), 42–43
self-assessment for, 53–55
sleep apnea, 15–16, 36–38
valvular heart disease, 40–41
treatment for, 177–78, 180–81

early detection and intervention, 85–86
multidisciplinary approach, 159, 181
multitiered approach, 84–85
rate-control strategy, 87–110
realistic expectations, 84–85, 180
rhythm-control strategy, 87–88, 110–14
stroke-prevention strategy, 113–16
triggers for, 43–51, 52*f*, 176
  alcohol, 43–44
  caffeine, 44
  dehydration, 46
  eating, 51
  electrolyte deficiencies, 44–46
  exercise, 49–50
  perfect storm of, 51–52
  poor sleep hygiene, 47–48
  self-assessment for, 56–58
  stress, 48–49
  time of day, 50
  types of, xiv–xv, 27, 29–31, 31*f*, 176
atrial flutter, 23, 191
  analogies, 24, 28*f*
  case studies, 26–27, 188
  circuit, 28*f*
  pacemakers, 94
  post-ablation, 109
atrial refractory period, 37, 42, 93
atrial tachycardia, 25, 109, 129, 148
AtriClip, 115, 116*f*
atrioventricular (AV) block, 120, 124, 133
atrioventricular (AV) node, 18, 19*f*, 21, 27, 145, 193
atrioventricular (AV) node ablation and pacemaker, 87–88, 94, 97, 113, 124
  blood thinners, 98
  eliminating need for rate-control medications, 100
  leadless pacemakers, 100
  overview of, 98, 99*f*, 100
automatic atrial tachycardia, 25
automaticity and automaticity arrhythmias, 24–25, 25*f*
automatic ventricular tachycardia, 25

autonomic nervous system (ANS), 18, 48, 138, 140, 144, 147, 181
AV (atrioventricular) block, 120, 124, 133
AV (atrioventricular) node, 18, 19*f*, 21, 27, 145, 193
AV node ablation and pacemaker. *See* atrioventricular node ablation and pacemaker

B

Bachmann's bundle, 19*f*
Berman, Marc, 149
beta-blockers, 35, 40, 49, 91, 100, 110, 111*t*, 112, 118–20, 184, 189
Betapace (sotalol), 89*t*, 90–91, 120–21
Biosense Webster, Inc., 171
BIOTRONIK, 128
Bird, Larry, 9
biventricular pacemakers, 96*f*, 113, 123–25
Blackburn, Elizabeth, 141
blood flow, 17*f*
  coronary artery disease and, 39–40
  dehydration and, 46
  diabetes and, 39
blood pressure, 124
  adrenaline and, 138
  exercise and, 50
  mindfulness and, 140
  music and, 150–51
  obesity and, 34
  rate-control medications and, 112, 119
  as risk factor and trigger, 35–36
  sleep and, 152
  sleep hygiene and, 47
  stress management and, 49
  yoga and, 148
blood thinners (anticoagulants), 73–74, 98, 113, 115, 132
blood urea nitrogen to creatinine ratio (BUN/Cr), 46
Boston Scientific, 128
Boston University, 34
bradycardia, 18
brain-heart connection, 144–45, 181

autonomic nervous system, 144
heart as representation of connection
to others, 144–45
"mind," 144
"organic brain," 144
BUN/Cr (blood urea nitrogen to creatinine ratio), 46
bundle branch block, 125
bundle of His, 19*f*
Bystolic (nebivolol), 35, 111*t*, 112

C

CAD (coronary artery disease; atherosclerosis), 32, 39–40, 90–91,
119–20, 124, 189
caffeine
insomnia and, 47
reducing, 35, 42
as trigger, 44
calcium channel blockers, 24, 35–36,
100, 111*t*, 112, 118–19
Calm app, 141, 146–47
Campbell, Joseph, 179
carbohydrates, 151
cardiac ablation, 98–110, 129–33, 177,
181
for atrial flutter, 26–27, 28*f*
AV node ablation, 98, 99*f*, 100
case studies, 64, 184, 186–90
in combination with other treatments,
30
compared to other treatments, 122
defined, xv, 129
epicardial fat and, 34–35
factors influencing success of, 85
individualized treatment, 130
left atrial ablation, 100–101, 102*f–3f*,
104, 105*f*, 106, 107*f–8f*, 109–10
post-procedure, 132
procedures for, 130–31
rate-control *vs.* rhythm-control strategy, 87–88
recurrent AFib, 130, 132
reentrant arrhythmias, 24
risks, 133
success rate, 133

types of, 104, 105*f*, 106, 129
cardiac conduction system, 18–20, 19*f*
autonomic nervous system, 18
AV node, 18, 19*f*
Bachmann's bundle, 19*f*
bradycardia, 18
bundle of His, 19*f*
causes of cardiac arrhythmias, 23–25,
25*f*
EKG components, 20*f*, 21
ion channel receptors, 21, 22*f*, 23
left bundle branch, 19*f*, 20
left ventricle, 20
Purkinje fibers, 19*f*
right bundle branch, 19*f*, 20
right ventricle, 20
sinus node, 18, 19*f*
tachycardia, 18
cardiac electrophysiologists (EPs),
157–58
characteristics of, 158
defined, xiv, 194
finding, 158
cardiac tamponade, 133
Cardiovascular Research, 45
cardioversion, xv, 46, 49, 61, 92*f*, 177,
190
case study, 63–64
clarifying source of symptoms, 91
compared to other treatments, 122
defined, 91
success rate, 91, 93
carvedilol (Coreg), 35, 111*t*, 112
case studies
Brenda (atrial flutter), 26–27
Chris (AFib), 8, 184–85
Eric (paroxysmal AFib and sleep
apnea), 15–16
Jack (AFib patient), 86, 189–91
Joe (persistent AFib), 63–64
Johnny (AFib), 51
Kelsey (AFib), 8, 185–87
Mitch (long-standing persistent AFib
and sleep apnea), 38
Pat (AFib), 9, 188–89
Sean (AFib), 51
Susan (AFib), 52

Tom (AFib), 8–9, 187–88
catecholamine, 138
central sleep apnea, 36
CFAE (complex fractionated atrial electrogram ablation), 106, 109
CHA_2DS_2-VAS_2 screening, 114*f*
Checklist Manifesto, The (Gawande), xvii
CHF. *See* congestive heart failure
chordae tendinae, 17*f*
classical music, 150–51
codes, 5
complex fractionated atrial electrogram ablation (CFAE), 106, 109
computed tomography (CT), 104, 131
concealed accessory pathways, 185
Confucius, 143
congestive heart failure (CHF), xv–xvi, 31, 84, 90–91, 110, 112, 121–22, 125, 142, 181
  case study, 38
  defined, 194
  as risk factor and trigger, 40
  types of, 40
continuous positive airway pressure (CPAP), 16, 37–38
Convergent Procedure, 109, 115, 177
Coreg (carvedilol), 35, 111*t*, 112
coronary artery disease (CAD; atherosclerosis), 32, 39–40, 90–91, 119–20, 124, 189
coronary sinus, 29, 104
cortisol
  mindfulness and, 140
  music and, 150
  sleep hygiene and, 47
Coumadin (warfarin), 113, 115
Cousins, Norman, 154
Cox, James, 41
CPAP (continuous positive airway pressure), 16, 37–38
cryoballoon ablation, 64, 104, 105*f*, 106, 129, 177, 186
CT (computed tomography), 104, 131
CTI (cavo-tricuspid isthmus) flutter line, 106

D

dabigatran (Pradaxa), 115
deep breathing, 48, 139–40
defibrillators, implantable, 125, 166
dehydration, 46
dementia, xvi, 63, 109, 115
Desai, Aseem
  diagnosis and management of personal medical problem, 3–4, 7
  father's health crisis and death, 1–3, 7, 158
  mother's health crisis and death, 4–7
diabetes
  case study, 9, 188
  nutrition and, 151
  obesity and, 34
  as risk factor, 32, 39, 176
  sick sinus syndrome and, 124
diastolic congestive heart failure, 40
digoxin, 100, 111*t*, 112
dihydropyridine, 35
diltiazem, 35, 111*t*, 112, 118, 187–88
disopyramide (Norpace), 89*t*, 120
Doctor's Best, 45
dofetilide (Tikosyn), 89*t*, 90–91, 120–21, 189–90
dronedarone (Multaq), 89*t*, 90–91, 120–22, 189
dual-chamber pacemakers, 94, 95*f*, 123–24

E

Earhart, Amelia, 83
eating, as trigger, 51
ECG app, 26
echocardiography (ultrasonography), 62, 91, 131
edoxaban (Savaysa), 115
ejection fraction, 112
electrocardiography (EKG), 20*f*, 21, 176
  antiarrhythmic drugs and, 120
  diagnosis of AFib, 60–62, 66
  PR interval, 20*f*, 21
  P wave, 20*f*, 21
  QRS complex, 20*f*, 21
  QT interval, 20*f*, 21

T wave, 20*f*, 21
electrolyte deficiencies
    dehydration and, 46
    as trigger, 44–46
electrophysiologists. *See* cardiac
    electrophysiologists
electrophysiology studies (EPS), 194
Eliquis (apixaban), 115
endorphins, 42, 147
epicardial fat, 34
EPs. *See* cardiac electrophysiologists
EPS (electrophysiology studies), 194
event recorders, 165
    compared to other monitors, 66
    image of, 70*f*
    insurance coverage, 69
    overview of, 80*f*
    utility of, 69
exercise, 35, 42, 147–49
    athleticism as risk factor, 41–42
    benefits of, 147–48
    insomnia and, 47
    as trigger, 49–50, 148
    yoga, 148–49

F

family
    detection of symptoms, 61–64
    keeping informed of your health, 6–7
    social support system, 152–53, 159
FDA, 75, 164–65
fight-or-flight response, 138, 144
FIRE and ICE Trial, 104
flecainide (Tambocor), 89*t*, 90, 119–22,
    184
Foley catheters, 131
Framingham Heart Study, 32, 34

G

gamma-aminobutyric acid (GABA)
    modifiers, 47
Gawande, Atul, xvii
genetics
    nature and nurture, 16, 18, 32
    as risk factor, 32
getsmartaboutafib.com, 171
ginger, 152

grounding, 149

H

Haïssaguerre, Michel, 100
HAS-BLED screening, 114*f*
Headspace app, 141, 147
health care team, 153, 157–59
    "AFib clinics," 159, 181
    allied health professionals, 158–59
    cardiac electrophysiologists (EPs),
        157–58
    finding specialists, 158, 170–72
    mass education of health care profes-
        sionals, 86, 181
    questions to ask specialist, 81–82
    social support system, 159
    team-based care, 158–59
Health Insurance Portability and
    Accounting Act (HIPAA), 183
heart
    anatomy of, 17*f*, 18
    blood flow in, 17*f*
    brain-heart connection, 144–45, 181
    cardiac conduction system, 18–20, 19*f*
    heart attack, 2, 23, 40, 48, 62, 126,
        133, 194
heartbeats
    effect on ion channel receptors, 22*f*, 23
    EKG components, 20*f*, 21
    electrical process of, 18, 20
HeartMath, 142
heart-rhythm monitoring, 65–66,
    163–66
    importance of, 163–64
    insurance coverage, 69
    Kardia device, 164
    pacemakers and defibrillators, 166
    types of monitors, 42, 66–80, 164–66,
        176, 186–89
Heart Rhythm Society, 158
Hills, Mellanie True, 170
HIPAA (Health Insurance Portability
    and Accounting Act), 183
Hippocrates, 151
Hirsch, Edward, 1
Holter monitors, 42, 67–68, 165, 176
    compared to other monitors, 66
    image of, 67*f*

insurance coverage, 69
  overview of, 80*f*
  utility of, 68
hypnosis, 147
hypoxia, 37

I

ibutilide, 122
idiopathic ventricular tachycardia, 24
implantable loop monitors, 166, 176,
      189
  case study, 187
  compared to other monitors, 66
  image of, 76*f*
  overview of, 80*f*
  utility of, 75–77
Inderol (propranolol), 35, 111*t*, 112
inferior vena cava, 17*f*
Insight Timer app, 141
insomnia, 47
insurance coverage, 118
interventricular septum, 17*f*
iodine, 91, 120
ion channel receptors
  analogy describing, 21, 22*f*, 23
  effect of heartbeat on, 22*f*, 23
  effects of antiarrhythmic drugs, 23
isoproterenol (adrenaline), 101

J

Jansen, Kenley, 1
journaling, 47
Journal of the American College of
      Cardiology, 148

K

Kabat-Zinn, Jon, 140
Kardia device, 77, 164, 186
Keller, Helen, xiii
King, Billie Jean, 157

L

Lakkireddy, Dhanunjaya, 148
Lariat Procedure, 115, 116*f*
laughter, 154

leadless pacemakers, 96*f*, 97–98, 100,
      113, 123–24, 128, 177
left atrial ablation, 102*f*–3*f*, 104, 105*f*,
      106, 107*f*–8*f*, 109–10
  pulmonary vein isolation, 100–101,
      109
  recurrent AFib, 104
  scarring and success rates, 109
  3-D electroanatomic mapping, 101,
      102*f*–3*f*
left atrial appendage, 29, 104
left atrial appendage ligation, 115
left atrial appendage occlusion, 98, 115,
      116*f*
left atrial-esophageal fistula, 133
left atrial posterior wall isolation (PWI),
      64, 106
left atrial roof line, 106
left atrium, 17*f*
  high blood pressure and, 35
  size and volume of, 62
  valvular heart disease, 41
left bundle branch, 19*f*, 20
left pulmonary veins, 17*f*, 29
left ventricle, 17*f*, 20
ligament of Marshall, 29, 104
Locke, John, 15
Lombardi, Vince, 157
long-standing persistent atrial
      fibrillation
  cardiac ablation success rate, 133
  case study, 38
  defined, 30, 31*f*, 176, 194
Lopressor (metoprolol; Toprol), 35,
      111*t*, 112, 118, 184, 187–88

M

Madsen, Karsten, 83
magnesium supplementation, 35, 42,
      44–45
  foods high in magnesium, 151
  for insomnia, 47
  intravenous, 45–46
  before sleep, 152
  types of, 45
magnetic resonance imaging (MRI),
      62–63, 109
Maimonides, 59

Mandel, Howie, 59
Manilow, Barry, 163
maze procedure, 41
meditation, 140–41
Mediterranean diet, 151
Medtronic, 128
melatonin, 47
metoprolol (Toprol; Lopressor), 35,
    111*t*, 112, 118, 184, 187–88
mindfulness, 47–49, 140–41, 146–47
Mindfulness-Based Stress Reduction
    program, 140
mitral valve, 17*f*
MRI (magnetic resonance imaging),
    62–63, 109
Multaq (dronedarone), 89*t*, 90–91,
    120–22, 189
music, 150–51
myocardium, 17*f*

N

National Heart, Lung, and Blood Insti-
    tute, 34
Natural Vitality Calm Gummies, 45
nature, 149
Nealon, Kevin, 143
nebivolol (Bystolic), 35, 111*t*, 112
New England Journal of Medicine, 100
Nietzsche, Friedrich, xiii
nondihydropyridine, 35–36
normal sinus rhythm, xiii, 194
Norpace (disopyramide), 89*t*, 120
Northwestern University, 2
Novoa, Roberto, 147
nutrition, 151–52

O

obesity, 124
    nutrition and, 152
    as risk factor, 34–35
    sleep apnea and, 36
obstructive sleep apnea (OSA), 36, 38
orthodromic reciprocating tachycardia,
    185

P

pacemakers, 60, 93–94, 95*f*–96*f*, 97–98,
    122–28, 177
    algorithm to suppress PACs, 93
    antitachycardia pacing, 94
    AV node ablation and, 87–88, 94,
        97–98, 99*f*, 100, 113, 124
    battery changes, 123
    battery life, 127–28
    brands of, 128
    capture threshold, 126
    case study, 191
    in combination with medication, 93
    in combination with other treatments,
        30
    compared to other treatments, 122
    defined, 123, 194
    frequency of evaluation, 127
    lead impedance, 126
    limitations after procedure, 127
    parts of, 123
    procedures for, 125–26
    reasons for using, 124–25
    restrictions after procedure, 128
    risks, 126
    types of, 94–98, 100, 113, 123–25,
        128, 177
    using as monitor, 166
Pacerone (amiodarone), 89*t*, 90–91,
    120–22, 189
PACs. *See* premature atrial contractions
PAF. *See* paroxysmal atrial fibrillation
panic/anxiety attacks, 60, 65
papillary muscles, 17*f*
parasympathetic ganglionic plexi, 140
parasympathetic nervous system (PNS),
    41, 50–51, 120, 138, 144
paroxysmal atrial fibrillation (PAF)
    cardiac ablation success rate, 133
    defined, xiv, 29, 31*f*, 176, 194
    defining success in overcoming, 84
    diagnosis of, 59–60, 65
    left atrial ablation, 100, 104, 109
patch monitors, 67–68, 166, 176
    case study, 186
    compared to other monitors, 66
    image of, 74*f*

insurance coverage, 69
  overview of, 80f
  utility of, 73–74
pericarditis, 132–33
permanent atrial fibrillation, xv, 29
  AV node ablation, 100
  as decision rather than mechanism,
    30, 31f
  defined, 176, 195
  defining success in overcoming, 84
persistent atrial fibrillation
  cardiac ablation success rate, 133
  case study, 63–64, 190
  defined, xiv–xv, 29–30, 31f, 176, 195
  defining success in overcoming, 84
  diagnosis of, 60–62
  left atrial ablation, 106, 109
phrenic nerve, 106
phrenic nerve paralysis, 133
PNS (parasympathetic nervous system),
    41, 50–51, 120, 138, 144
post-conversion pauses, 190–91
posterior wall, 29, 104
potassium channel blockers, 89t, 90–91.
    See also names of specific drugs
potassium, foods high in, 151
Pradaxa (dabigatran), 115
premature atrial contractions (PACs),
    25, 100–101, 110
  athleticism and AFib, 41–42
  defined, 195
  exercise and, 148
  pacemakers, 93
  as risk factor and trigger, 42–43
  telemetry monitors, 72
premature ventricular contraction
    (PVC) cardiomyopathy, 68
premature ventricular contractions
    (PVCs), 25, 45, 65–66
  Holter monitors, 68
  telemetry monitors, 72
Presley, Elvis, 169
proarrhythmic drugs, 88, 120–21, 187
procainamide, 120
propafenone (Rhythmol), 89t, 90,
    119–22
propranolol (Inderol), 35, 111t, 112

pulmonary trunk, 17f
pulmonary vein isolation, 100–101, 109
pulmonary veins, 101, 195
pulmonary vein stenosis, 133
pulmonic valve, 17f
Purkinje fibers, 19f
PVC cardiomyopathy, 68
PVCs. See premature ventricular
    contractions
PWI (left atrial posterior wall isolation),
    64, 106
Pyridium, 131

Q

quinidine, 120

R

radiofrequency (RF) ablation, 64, 104,
    105f, 106, 113, 177, 187
rate-control medications, 110, 111t,
    112, 177
  beta-blockers, 110, 111t, 112, 118–19
  calcium channel blockers, 112,
    118–19
  eliminating need for with AV node
    ablation and pacemaker, 100
  side effects of, 119
rate-control strategies, 87–88, 110–14
  AV node ablation and pacemaker, 94,
    97, 113
  medications, 110, 111t, 112, 118–19
  pacemakers, 94, 97
recurrent atrial fibrillation, 34, 39, 87,
    130, 132, 177
reentry and reentrant arrhythmias
  case study, 26–27
  defined, 23–24, 25f, 195
  premature atrial contractions and, 42
regurgitation, 41
remote/robotic magnetic ablation, 106,
    129
RF (radiofrequency) ablation, 64, 104,
    105f, 106, 113, 177, 187
rhythm-control strategies, 87–110
  antiarrhythmic drugs, 88, 89t, 90–91,
    119–21

cardiac ablation, 98–110
cardioversion, 91, 92*f,* 93
pacemakers, 93–94, 95*f*–96*f,* 97–98
Rhythmol (propafenone), 89*t,* 90,
     119–22
right atrial cavo-tricuspid isthmus (CTI)
     flutter line, 106
right atrium, 17*f,* 41
right bundle branch, 19*f,* 20
right pulmonary veins, 17*f,* 29
right ventricle, 17*f,* 20
Rim, J. R., 181
rivaroxaban (Xarelto), 115
Ruhr-University Bochum, 150

S

salt, 35, 151
saturated fats, 151
Savaysa (edoxaban), 115
self-assessments
     risk factors for AFib, 53–55
     triggers for AFib, 56–58
serotonin, 149
serotonin modifiers, 47
Shakespeare, William, 175
sick sinus syndrome, 93, 120, 124
silent AFib (asymptomatic episodes), 60,
     66, 69, 72, 75, 166, 187
Simmons, Gene, 137
Simple Habit app, 141
single-chamber pacemakers, 95*f,*
     123–24
sinus node (sinoatrial [SA] node), xiii,
     18, 19*f,* 145, 195
sinus rhythm
     defined, xiii
     "sinus rhythm begets sinus rhythm,"
         39, 51, 177–78
     size of left atrium and, 62
     success in treatment of AFib, xv, 39
sleep apnea, 124
     case study, 15–16, 38
     causes of, 36
     CPAP, 16, 37–38
     as risk factor, 36–38
     screening for, 37
     symptoms of, 36

treatment for, 16, 37–38
sleep hygiene, 152
     heart attacks and, 48
     insomnia, 47
     poor, as trigger, 47–48
smartphone-enabled and smartwatch
     monitors, 66, 77, 78*f,* 79, 80*f,* 164,
     176
social support system, 152–53, 159
sodium channel blockers, 89*t,* 90. *See
     also names of specific drugs*
sotalol (Betapace), 89*t,* 90–91, 120–21
Sprouts, 45
Stanford University, 165
Stanford University Medical Center, 3
stenosis, 41
Still the Mind (Watts), 49
stopafib.org, 159, 186
stress
     stress management, 42–43, 48–49,
         140–42
     time of day and, 50
     as trigger, 48–49
stress hormones, 47, 140, 147, 152
stroke, xv–xvi, 31, 73–74, 87, 133, 171
     age and, 32
     diabetes and, 39
     risk of by age, 32, 34
     of unknown origin (cryptogenic), 66
stroke-prevention strategy, 84, 113–16
     blood thinners, 113, 115, 116*f*
     left atrial appendage occlusion, 115,
         116*f*
     screening, 114*f*
     stylets, 126
subcutaneous implantable monitors. *See*
     implantable loop monitors
sunlight, 149
superior vena cava (SVC), 17*f,* 29, 104,
     188
supraventricular tachycardia (SVT), 23,
     29, 60, 184–85
sympathetic nervous system, 50, 138,
     144
symptomatic bradycardia, 124
syncope, 77
systolic congestive heart failure, 40

T

tachycardia, 18
tachycardia-bradycardia syndrome, 93, 124
tachycardia cardiomyopathy, 164
tachycardia mediated cardiomyopathy, 68
Tambocor (flecainide), 89*t*, 90, 119–22, 184
TED talks, 48
telemetry monitors, 71–73, 165, 176
  case study, 188
  compared to other monitors, 66
  image of, 71*f*
  insurance coverage, 69
  overview of, 80*f*
  utility of, 72–73
telomerase, 141
telomeres, 141
Tenormin (atenolol), 35, 111*t*, 112, 118
3-D electroanatomic mapping, 101, 102*f*–3*f*
TIA (transient ischemic attack), 133
Tikosyn (dofetilide), 89*t*, 90–91, 120–21, 189–90
time of day, as trigger, 50
Tolle, Eckhart, 137
toolbox concept, 145–54
  exercise, 147–49
  health care team, 153
  laughter, 154
  mindfulness, 146–47
  music, 150–51
  nature, 149
  nutrition, 151–52
  sleep, 152
  social support system, 152–53
Toprol (metoprolol; Lopressor), 35, 111*t*, 112, 118, 184, 187–88
torsades de pointes, 91, 121
transient ischemic attack (TIA), 133
Trappe, H. J., 150
tricuspid valve, 17*f*
triggered activity and triggered activity arrhythmias, 24, 25*f*
tryptophan, 47
turmeric, 152

U

ultrasonography (echocardiography), 62, 91, 131
University of California, San Francisco, 42
University of Michigan, 149
University of Utah, 109

V

vagally triggered atrial fibrillation, 50–51
Valentine's Day, 145
valvular heart disease, 40–41
venography, 125
ventricular tachycardia, 23–25, 45
verapamil, 35, 111*t*, 112
vitamin D, 149

W

Walker, Matt, 48
warfarin (Coumadin), 113, 115
Watchman Procedure, 115, 116*f*
water intake, 44, 46
Watts, Alan, 49
Wolff-Parkinson-White syndrome, 23, 29

X

Xarelto (rivaroxaban), 115

Y

yoga, 148–49
YouTube, 147

Z

Zubeldia, Haimar, 169

Notes

About the Author

Dr. Aseem Desai is a cardiac electrophysiologist (EP), a physician specializing in heart rhythm disorders. He has been caring for people with atrial fibrillation (AFib) for over seventeen years and currently practices in Orange County, California. Dr. Desai graduated from Northwestern University Medical School as part of the Honors Program in Medical Education (HPME). He did his internship, residency, chief residency, cardiology fellowship, and electrophysiology fellowship at Stanford University Medical Center. Dr. Desai served as Assistant Professor of Medicine and Director of Implantable Device Therapy at the University of Chicago Hospital. As an author of several scientific manuscripts, he has published in peer-reviewed journals such as *HeartRhythm Journal, Journal of the American College of Cardiology, American Journal of Medicine*, and *Annals of Internal Medicine*. Dr. Desai's passion for connecting with people has allowed him to increase AFib awareness through speaking engagements, writing for the general public on blogs such as *The Doctor Weighs In,* and on his YouTube channel, which features educational and human-interest stories. He provides personalized care based on the statement: "Doctor, if I were a family member of yours, what would you recommend?" When he's not helping patients, he enjoys spending time with his family, singing, playing guitar, reading, and yoga.